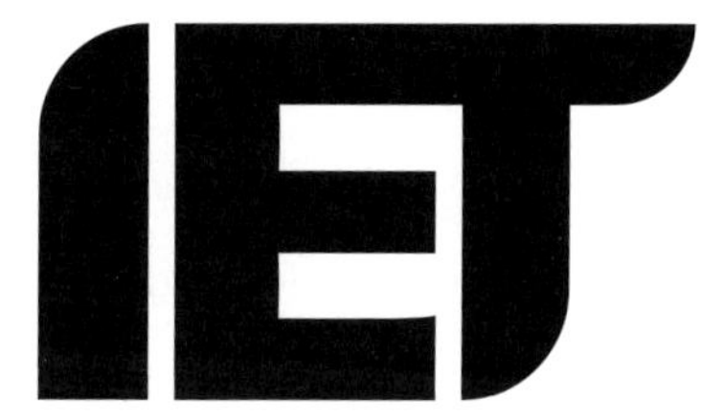

GUIDE TO ELECTRICAL INSTALLATIONS IN MEDICAL LOCATIONS

Published by The Institution of Engineering and Technology, London, United Kingdom

The Institution of Engineering and Technology is registered as a Charity in England & Wales (no. 211014) and Scotland (no. SC038698).

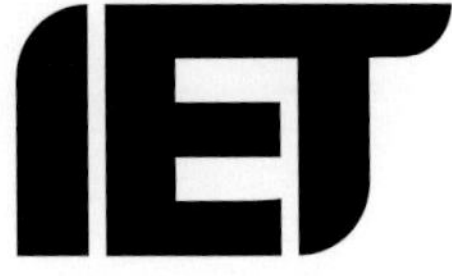

The Institution of Engineering and Technology is the institution formed by the joining together of the IEE (The Institution of Electrical Engineers) and the IIE (The Institution of Incorporated Engineers). The new Institution is the inheritor of the IEE brand and all its products and services, such as this one, which we hope you find useful.

First published 2017

Copies of this publication may be obtained from:
The Institution of Engineering and Technology
PO Box 96, Stevenage, SG1 2SD, UK
Tel: +44 (0)1438 767328
Email: sales@theiet.org
www.electrical.theiet.org/books

ISBN 978-1-84919-767-0 (paperback)
ISBN 978-1-84919-768-7 (electronic)

Typeset in the UK by the Institution of Engineering and Technology, Stevenage
Printed and bound in the UK by Sterling Press Ltd, Kettering

Contents

A Guide to Electrical Installations in Medical Locations
© The Institution of Engineering and Technology

About the author

I am an experienced Chartered Engineer and I still learn something new every single day. After the first three months of my apprenticeship, I thought I had all the information I needed for the rest of my electrical career, and there was nothing more to learn. I hadn't heard of unconscious incompetence then. I know now it is a stage where we are at our most vulnerable.

Armed with my three months' electrical training and four weeks' day release, I got on with the job and soon understood that I didn't know everything. I developed a passion for always learning more. During the final phases of my formal apprenticeship, the electrical industry was turned upside down by the introduction of the 15th Edition of BS 7671. I realised at that point that most engineers are just 'experienced apprentices', trying to adapt and keep up with an ever-changing and developing industry.

The 15th Edition brought about practices that, to me at the time, seemed incorrect, unnecessary and the stuff of myths and legends. As a fledgling electrician I challenged the practice, but chose the wrong forum, so my concerns fell on deaf ears. However, as time progressed, requirements were changed and guidance was issued, the mythical requirements became clearer and their rationale made more sense.

My aim since then has been to demystify industry practices where I have the ability to do so. Where possible and as far as practicable, I try to address misunderstanding and improve knowledge and skills to rule out errors built into folklore practices. The excuse 'we did this on the last five jobs so it must be right' isn't always right, especially where there is no foundation for what is being done.

The electrical industry that serves the medical industry suffers many misunderstandings and is the subject of many myths of what can be done, what can't be done and what will seriously injure a patient. These myths can be attributed to the misapplication and misunderstanding of installation and equipment standards.

Guide to Electrical Installations for Medical Locations aims to demystify and improve understanding. It intends to bridge a gap in knowledge and application to improve electrical standards and installation delivery – the outcomes of which must have, however indirect, a positive effect on patient well-being.

Acknowledgements

I would like to send a special thank you to my friends and colleagues including Michael Bernard, who has been a tremendous help with some of the particularly difficult sections of this Guide, Mohamed Al Rufaie for his support and review work and thanks to the numerous other industry professionals and contributors who are too many to name.

I would like to thank my wife Carol and the rest of my family for putting up with me during the writing stage. I would also like to give a special acknowledgement to my daughter Victoria, the most energetic enthusiastic person I have ever met, sadly she never got to see it published, I want to say – I finally got there Vic!

Foreword

Application of this guidance

This Guide aims to assist the reader when working through the requirements for medical locations, which, regardless of experience, can prove to be daunting at times. This Guide also explains the requirements of BS 7671 that relate to medical locations. It provides support through scenarios to give readers, including experienced engineers, the confidence to apply this guidance with their skill and judgement and, in so doing, to satisfy the electrical requirements.

History of Section 710

Section 710 was first published in BS 7671:2008(2011) and was based on a draft international Harmonized Document (HD) 60364-7-710, which, in the fullness of time, was eventually agreed by all EU member states in April 2012 as HD 60364-7-710:2012. The requirements of Section 710 in BS 7671:2008(2011) were far more onerous than the requirements set out in the finalised HD.

As a result of these differences in May 2013 JPEL/64, the Committee that oversees the technical content of BS 7671, took the unprecedented step to issue a full section corrigendum in order to clarify a number of points on medical locations design. The corrigendum brought the UK back into line with the technical intent of HD 60364-7-710:2012.

Validity of information

Special locations are covered generally by the IET publication Guidance Note 7, which gives an IET commentary and viewpoint on the special locations contained within BS 7671. With the modification of Section 710 issued in the June 2013 corrigendum, a large amount of the guidance within Chapter 9 of that book became outdated.

Amendment No. 3 (2015) to BS 7671:2008 (BS 7671:2008+A3:2015) was issued in January 2015 and required any designs started after 30 June 2015 to comply with this new amendment.

As Section 710 was amended in 2013, there are only minor changes to Section 710; however, changes within the main document have an effect on medical location design, therefore caution is advised in reading only Section 710.

Following publication of BS 7671:2008+A3:2015, Guidance Note 7 (Chapter 9 Medical Locations) has been updated and republished. The information contained within Guidance Note 7 is a commentary on the Wiring Regulations and is fully aligned with the theories presented in this Guide.

This Guide is provided to enable designers, maintainers and contractors to better understand electrical installations for medical locations and assist with cutting through the myths and 'black art' culture, which has developed over the past few years.

References to Health Technical Memorandum (HTM) or Health Building Notes (HBNs) etc. are deemed to include the relevant standard for the particular home country in the United Kingdom, for example, for Scotland, Scottish Health Technical Memorandums (SHTMs) are applicable.

It must be noted that, although out of date in many areas, the HTMs and HBNs form the backbone of healthcare design practice. Designers and installers and those inspecting these hospital installations are required to have an understanding of these documents in order to understand healthcare design philosophy, which is outside the scope of any one publication. Simple examples of this would be the link between the operational elements of Progressive Horizontal Evacuation (moving patients from one area to another without leaving the building), structural fire precautions, ventilation, and fire alarm requirements. All of these subject areas cover different disciplines and also interface with the electrical systems, however, they cannot all be contained in one publication.

Introduction 1

This Guide has been produced to support engineers who are involved in the design, construction and inspection and testing of electrical installations in medical locations. It provides background information and details to allow informed decisions to be made. The guidance is not meant to be prescriptive or restrictive. It aims to guide the reader through process, adding clarity to the information that is currently available or specified as part of a contract.

Unlike many other engineering guides, this guidance centres on the needs of the patient within a clinical environment. It will assist the reader to produce better solutions by concentrating on the needs of the patient and the clinicians that provide patient care.

1.1 Special location information

BS 7671:2008+A3:2015 contains 19 special locations, of which Section 710 Medical Locations is one. The recurring theme of all special location guidance is that the special location requirements are not stand-alone documents; they have to be read in conjunction with the main body of the requirements of BS 7671.

The general requirements contained in the main body of BS 7671 are applicable to all electrical installations. The specific requirements of a special location are provided to supplement or modify the general requirements to be applicable to the particular special location.

1.2 Who is Section 710 applicable to?

Section 710 is part of the national standard for electrical installations, so it is applicable across the UK and any other states or countries where BS 7671 is applied. The technical intent of Section 710 is derived from HD 60364-7-710:2012, which is the Harmonized Document (HD) for CENELEC countries. In turn, the HD 60364 series is based on the IEC 60364 series of standards published by the International Electrotechnical Commission (IEC).

CENELEC, which is the acronym for Comité Européen de Normalisation Électrotechnique (European Committee for Electrotechnical Standardization), is responsible for standardization in the electrotechnical engineering field.

Section 710 is therefore applicable to all persons involved in the design, construction, operation, maintenance (including periodic inspection) and eventual deconstruction of any medical location covered in the scope.

1.3   What type of installations does Section 710 cover?

The scope of Section 710 states that it applies to electrical installations in hospitals, private clinics, medical and dental practices, healthcare and dedicated medical rooms in the workplace and also for locations carrying out medical research.

The supporting notes suggest that the requirements of Section 710 could also be applied to veterinary surgeries. This requirement would, in most cases, be a 'nice to have' rather than a definite requirement. Specialist veterinary surgeries, for high value or rare animals, may have a more definite requirement than the general high street veterinary surgery.

Whilst Section 710 also applies to medical locations within mobile medical units, it is also important to understand that Section 717 Mobile or Transportable Units of BS 7671 also applies in that type of unit.

1.4   What is not covered by Section 710?

Medical electrical equipment is not covered by Section 710, as such items of equipment are covered by the BS EN 60601 series. However, this equipment cannot be ignored as it is integral to the use and purpose of a medical location and the treatment of the patient. Medical electrical equipment will therefore be discussed in appropriate sections of this Guide.

1.5   Background to Section 710

Section 710 is part of BS 7671 which is itself a standard, not a specification or a guidance document. Consequently, the language that is used is, as with all standards, one of regulatory requirements. These requirements stipulate criteria that need to be satisfied so that designers can discharge their duty in accordance with the requirements of the Electricity at Work Regulations 1989.

1.6 History

The IET Wiring Regulations (previously referred to as the IEE Wiring Regulations) have been in force since Victorian times with the first edition, issued in 1882, entitled *Rules and Regulations for the Prevention of Fire Risks Arising from Electric Lighting*. There have been a number of modifications since that time and in 1992 it became a British Standard.

▼ **Figure 1.1** First Edition, 1882

RULES AND REGULATIONS

FOR THE PREVENTION OF FIRE RISKS ARISING FROM ELECTRIC LIGHTING,

Recommended by the Council in accordance with the Report of the Committee appointed by them on May 11, 1882, to consider the subject.

MEMBERS OF THE COMMITTEE.

Professor W. G. Adams, F.R.S., *Vice-President.*	Professor D. E. Hughes, F.R.S., *Vice-President.*
Sir Charles T. Bright.	W. H. Preece, F.R.S., *Past President.*
T. Russell Crompton.	
R. E. Crompton.	Alexander Siemens.
W. Crookes, F.R.S.	C. E. Spagnoletti, *Vice-President.*
Warren De la Rue, D.C.L., F.R.S.	James N. Shoolbred.
Professor G. C. Foster, F.R.S., *Past President.*	Augustus Stroh.
Edward Graves.	Sir William Thomson, F.R.S., *Past President.*
J. E. H. Gordon.	Lieut.-Colonel C. E. Webber, R.E., *President.*
Dr. J. Hopkinson, F.R.S.	

These rules and regulations are drawn up not only for the guidance and instruction of those who have electric lighting apparatus installed on their premises, but for the reduction to a minimum of those risks of fire which are inherent to every system of artificial illumination.

The chief dangers of every new application of electricity arise mainly from ignorance and inexperience on the part of those who supply and fit up the requisite plant.

The difficulties that beset the electrical engineer are chiefly internal and invisible, and they can only be effectually guarded against by "testing," or probing with electric currents. They depend chiefly on leakage, undue resistance in the conductor, and bad joints, which lead to waste of energy and the production of heat. These defects can only be detected by measuring, by means of special apparatus, the currents that are either ordinarily or for

1.7 International Standards

International standards for the electrical industry are developed and published through the International Electrotechnical Commission (IEC). This body provides standards for all countries to use and, if required, to develop into their own standard.

The IEC 60364 series form a framework on which countries base their wiring rules and requirements. The documents are compiled and published as separate sections that relate to particular requirements.

In terms of medical locations, the original standard published by the International Electrotechnical Commission was IEC 60364-7-710:2002, which, for many years, was the reference point for medical locations in the UK beyond the information published by the Department of Health in their HTM series of documents.

Although published as an international standard, the fact remains that many IEC documents appear to have very little direct influence in the UK until they are adopted in CENELEC as HDs and, subsequently, included in UK standards such as BS 7671, or are expressly stated as a requirement in contract documents.

There were many delays in the inclusion of Section 710 into BS 7671. In order to fill the vacuum, IEC 60364-7-710:2002 was specified in many healthcare projects. Unfortunately, possibly due to a lack of understanding of the standard-setting process and hierarchy of the standards, many specifiers have continued to reference the document even though it has since been superseded by other publications.

1.8 Harmonization

Harmonization has been around longer than most engineers believe. Over recent years, British Standards have been harmonized with other European countries in CENELEC, which means that BS 7671 is based on both the International Standard IEC 60364 and the CENELEC HD 60364. Once an HD has been agreed across the member states of CENELEC each member state has to incorporate the technical intent of the specific HD into its own home standard, unless the detail within the HD conflicts with that country's statutory system or national laws.

This harmonization process ensures that international working is simplified and assists free trade between member countries, meaning that even though there may be national differences between member countries, a basic understanding of each other's requirements is retained.

1.9 HD 60364-7-710

Although there may be minor differences, fundamentally, the special locations are harmonized in terms of technical intent, as is the rest of BS 7671. Section 710 Medical Locations of BS 7671 is no different; this section is harmonized with the CENELEC Standard HD 60364-7-710:2012.

1.10 Longevity of information

Prior to the publication of this Guide, Amendment No. 3 (2015) of BS 7671:2008 was published and is referred to in this publication as BS 7671:2008+A3:2015.

As previously identified, special locations are not stand-alone documents, however, it should be noted that since the 2013 Corrigendum, only a small number of minor editorial modifications have been made directly to Section 710, although there are many changes to the general requirements which have a direct impact on electrical installations in medical locations.

1.11 International specifications

As Section 710 is based on the technical content of HD 60364-7-710, those using the standard may find an amount of similarity between this and other countries' national standards and requirements. However, if this guidance is used outside the UK, it is the reader's responsibility to check local regulations and requirements and to identify any changes to the HD that may or may not apply in that country.

▼ **Figure 1.2** Documents containing Section 710 Medical Locations

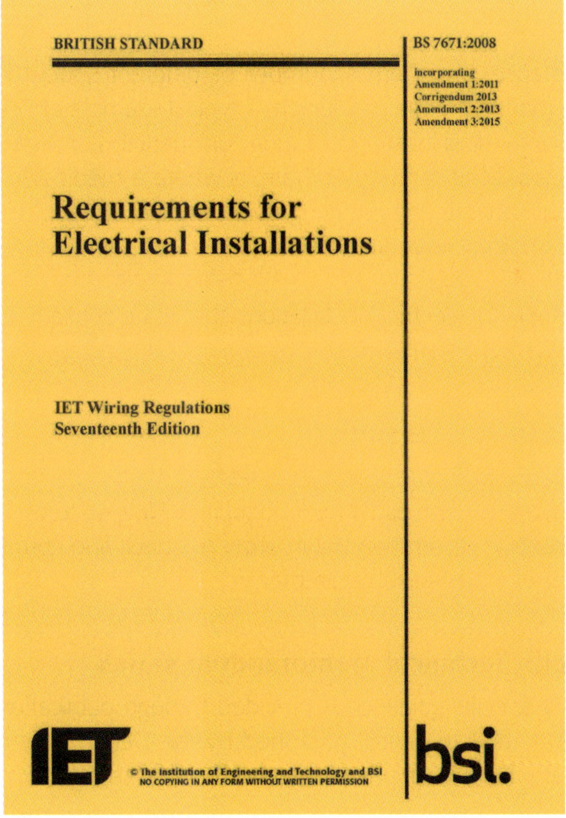

1.12   Reading material

This Guide is intended to be read in conjunction with BS 7671. As with BS 7671, it is virtually impossible to provide for every situation or eventuality. However, it is intended that the reader should be able to draw parallel circumstances and apply learning outcomes to other instances.

Where the design or installation of different medical applications is not specifically dealt with in this Guide, it is intended that the approach encouraged in this publication can assist the reader to apply the necessary requirements in order to meet the specific user or equipment requirements.

The approach should always be to assess the situation by first understanding what an area, building or installation will be used for. Once this is determined, the designer should refer to BS 7671.

1.12.1   BS 7671

As the national standard of the UK, BS 7671 has an overarching role in any system design and installation. Although Section 710 relates to medical locations, it must be remembered that the whole of the general requirements apply to an installation except where added to, or amended by, a particular special location requirement.

As a practising engineer, I often observe other engineers and sometimes have to check myself from falling into the trap of looking solely at Part 7 of BS 7671. A common example of this is the mistake of looking solely at Section 701 when carrying out a design in a bathroom instead of looking at the whole of the standard and then applying the additional requirements called for in the particular section.

In certain instances there are a number of different special locations that may be applicable to more than one installation. A typical example of this is where a bathroom is provided in a medical location requiring consideration of Sections 701 and 710. Less often encountered but certainly not rare, is where a medical location is provided in a mobile or transportable unit requiring consideration of Sections 717 and 710 and, of course, the usual general requirements.

The requirements for electrical installations should be applied as part of normal design processes.

1.12.2   Guidance Note suite

Most of the guidance for the general requirements within BS 7671 can be found within guidance documents such as the IET's Guidance Note suite of documents. The use of these documents is recommended in order to check and corroborate the individual's understanding of a particular requirement.

1.12.3   Health Technical Memorandum series

Other industry specific guidance is provided through publications such as the Health Technical Memorandum series, published by the Department of Health (DoH). This series looks at different aspects of healthcare engineering.

Historically, this series of documents provided up-to-date guidance and assurance by compliance with the particular document. However, as time has passed, many of these documents have not been updated alongside developments in methodology and standardisation, leaving certain elements of the documents within the series 'at odds' with current standards (as of the time of publication). It should be noted that these documents are absolutely healthcare focused and, despite their lack of update, still contain a wealth of information that is still valid or that can be applied to current design.

Consequently, where BS 7671 is silent on a matter, it is intended that other guidance, such as HTM 06-01 (Health Technical Memorandum 06-01 published by the DoH) or SHTM 06-01 for Scotland should be consulted. The application of any guidance material should not contradict the requirements of the national standard BS 7671.

It should be recognised that even specific electrical designs based on HTM and SHTM guidance have a wide remit in terms of health care installations. These design guides cannot necessarily focus on all matters relating to the design of a particular installation or scenario.

However, these publications are able to look at the wider implications of healthcare service delivery, for example, the business continuity and the wider impact of service delivery. A simple example of this is the fact that, although an operating theatre or other similar location may require a high level of resilience to maintain patient safety, the overall patient safety and 'experience' will be affected if ancillary services cannot be maintained, for instance, ancillary services such as cleaning and portering services. Business continuity is therefore an important factor in terms of overall healthcare provision.

This Guide should be used to assist in meeting the regulatory requirements of BS 7671, recognising that continuity of service provision is an important factor and looking to interpret service needs with technical and functional requirements of the standards and guidance. Consequently, this Guide encourages application of knowledge and understanding in conjunction with the national regulatory requirements of BS 7671. It encourages the designer to look at reasons for particular requirements to ensure that the design objectives are met.

A Guide to Electrical Installations in Medical Locations

Related reading 2

2.1 Definitions from Part 2 of BS 7671

There are numerous definitions set out in Part 2 of BS 7671:2008+A3:2015. A number of relevant definitions have been drawn out for 'ease of reference' as follows:

Medical location
Location intended for the purposes of diagnosis, treatment including cosmetic treatment, monitoring and care of patients.

Patient
Living being (person or animal) undergoing a medical, surgical or dental procedure.

> **Note:** A person under medical treatment for cosmetic purposes may be considered a patient.

Medical electrical equipment (ME equipment)
Electrical equipment having an applied part or transferring energy to or from the patient or detecting such energy transfer to or from the patient and which is:

(a) provided with not more than one connection to a particular supply mains, and
(b) intended by its manufacturer to be used
- in the diagnosis, treatment, or monitoring of a patient, or
- for compensation or alleviation of disease, injury or disability.

> **Note:** ME equipment includes those accessories as defined by the manufacturer that are necessary to enable the normal use of the ME equipment.

Applied part
Part of medical electrical equipment that in normal use necessarily comes into physical contact with the patient for ME equipment or an ME system to perform its function.

Group 0
Medical location where no applied parts are intended to be used and where discontinuity (failure) of the supply cannot cause danger to life.

Group 1
Medical location where discontinuity (failure) of the supply does not represent a threat to the safety of the patient and applied parts are intended to be used:
- externally
- invasively to any part of the body except where Group 2 applies.

Group 2

Medical location where applied parts are intended to be used, and where discontinuity (failure) of the supply can cause danger to life, in applications such as:

- intra-cardiac procedures
- vital treatments and surgical operations.

> **Note:** an intra-cardiac procedure is a procedure whereby an electrical conductor is placed within the heart of a patient or is likely to come into contact with the heart, such conductor being accessible outside the patient's body. In this context, an electrical conductor includes insulated wires such as cardiac pacing electrodes or intra-cardiac ECG electrodes, or insulated tubes filled with conducting fluids.

Medical electrical system (ME system)

Combination, as specified by the manufacturer, of items of equipment, at least one of which is medical electrical equipment to be interconnected by functional connection or by use of a multiple socket-outlet.

> **Note:** The system includes those accessories which are needed for operating the system and are specified by the manufacturer.

Medical IT system

IT electrical system fulfilling specific requirements for medical applications.

> **Note:** These supplies are also known as isolated power supply systems.

Patient environment

Any volume in which intentional or unintentional contact can occur between a patient and parts of the medical electrical equipment or medical electrical system or between a patient and other persons touching parts of the medical electrical equipment or medical electrical system.

2.2　Other terms not defined in Part 2 of BS 7671

▼ **Figure 2.1** Patient environment (BS EN 60601-1:2006)

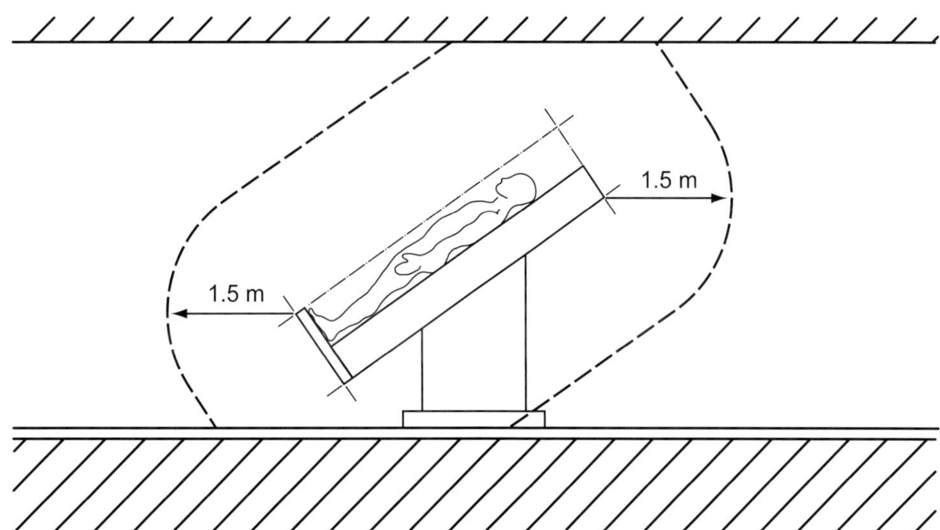

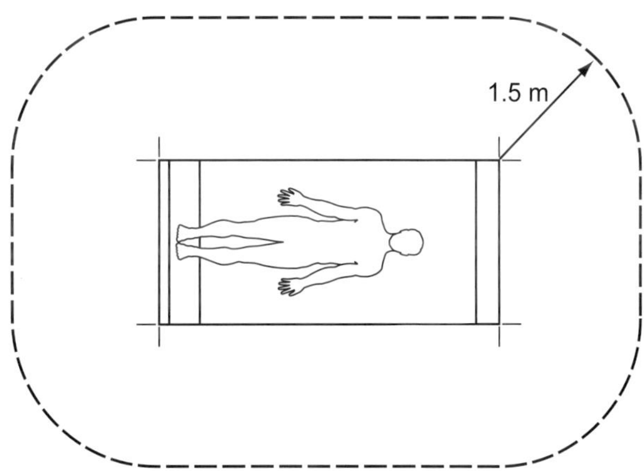

Note: the dimensions in the figure show the minimum extent of the patient environment in a free surrounding. It applies when the patient's position is pre-determined; if this is not achievable, all possible patient position should be considered.

Isolated Power Supply (IPS)

This is the term used as a descriptive term for a medical IT system. This system has been popularised in North America and is used extensively by manufacturers, designers, installers and client organisations in the UK.

Medical supply unit

Fixed equipment intended to supply electric power and/or medical gases and/or liquids and anaesthetic gas scavenging systems to medical areas of a health-care facility; see BS EN ISO 11197 for further information.

Note: medical supply units can include medical electrical equipment or medical electrical systems or parts thereof. Medical supply units can also consist of modular sections for electrical supply, lighting for therapy or illumination, communication, supply of medical gases and liquids, and anaesthetic gas scavenging systems. Some typical examples of medical supply units are bed head services modules, ceiling pendants, beams, booms, columns and pillars.

Touch current

Leakage current flowing from the enclosure or from parts thereof, excluding patient connections, accessible to any operator or patient in normal use, through an external path other than the protective earth conductor leading to earth or to another part of the enclosure.

> **Note:** the meaning of this term is the same as that of 'enclosure leakage current' in the first and second editions of BS EN 60601.

2.3 Associated regulations

2.3.1 Electricity at Work Regulations 1989

The Electricity at Work Regulations 1989 (EAWR) was introduced in association with the The Health and Safety at Work etc Act 1974 (the 'HASAWA'), which means that breaches in the EAWR will result in action being taken under HASAWA.

The EAWR came into force on 1st April 1990. The HASAWA imposes duties principally on employers, the self-employed and on employees, including certain classes of trainees. The EAWR imposes duties on people (referred to as 'duty-holders') in respect to systems, electrical equipment and conductors including work activities on or near electrical equipment. These duties are in addition to those imposed by the HASAWA.

The EAWR cover the principles of electrical safety that apply to work activities, the influence on those activities, systems of work, general selection of equipment, strength and integrity of electrical systems, isolation and safe systems and the competency of those working with electricity.

The Health and Safety Executive (HSE) publishes a memorandum of guidance, HSR 25, to assist designers, installers and duty-holders to understand the regulations and discharge their duties placed on them by the regulations.

2.3.2 Electricity Safety, Quality and Continuity Regulations 2002

The Electricity Safety, Quality and Continuity Regulations 2002, as amended (ESQCR) (SI 2002/2665) impose requirements for the installation and use of electric lines and apparatus of suppliers of electricity, including provisions for connections to earth. The safety aspects of the ESQCR are administered by the Health and Safety Executive.

The ESQCR places requirements, usually on supply companies or those associated with the supply of electricity, that are additional to those of the EAWR. Designers of installations have a responsibility to ensure that they meet the ESQCR.

2.3.3 Provision and Use of the Work Equipment Regulations 1998

The Provision and Use of Work Equipment Regulations 1998 (PUWER) is provided to ensure that work equipment is appropriate and safe to use.

PUWER Regulation 4 states:

(1) Every employer shall ensure that work equipment is so constructed or adapted as to be suitable for the purpose for which it is used or provided.

(2) In selecting work equipment, every employer shall have regard to the working conditions and to the risks to the health and safety of persons which exist in the premises or undertaking in which that work equipment is to be used and any additional risk posed by the use of that work equipment.

In terms of PUWER, 'work equipment' applies to any equipment, machinery, appliance, apparatus, tool or installation for use at work. This simply means that all equipment used in work places, including UK construction sites, must be fit for purpose and comply with the requirements by ensuring that the equipment used is suitable for the environment.

In all instances, those providing the equipment for use at work must take into account the additional risks involved in the particular use of that equipment within a specified location or environment.

For example, ME equipment is required to be maintained in accordance with BS EN 62353.

2.3.4   Construction Design and Management Regulations

Construction Design and Management Regulations 2015 (CDM 2015) came into force on 6th April 2015, replacing CDM 2007.

▼ **Figure 2.2** Construction Design and Management Regulations 2015 (image courtesy of HSE)

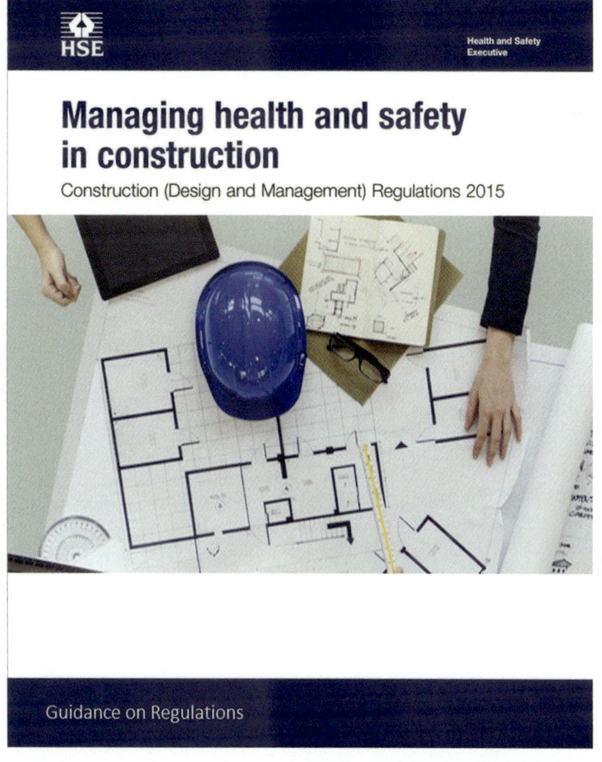

CDM 2015 is a key piece of construction safety legislation that levels accountability to all parties, including the client. Further advice is available on the HSE website.

2.4　BS 7671 and compliance with the Electricity at Work Regulations

BS 7671 is a British Standard, which is deemed by the HSE to be industry best practice. The HSE has a commentary in each edition of BS 7671, which for the current amendment states:

> *The Health and Safety Executive (HSE) welcomes the publication of BS 7671:2008, Requirements for Electrical Installations, IET (formerly IEE) Wiring Regulations 17th Edition, and its updating with the third amendment, published in 2015. BS 7671 and the IEE Wiring Regulations have been extensively referred to in HSE guidance over the years. Installations which conform to the standards laid down in BS 7671:2008+A3:2015 are regarded by HSE as likely to achieve conformity with the relevant parts of the Electricity at Work Regulations 1989. Existing installations may have been designed and installed to conform to the standards set by earlier editions of BS 7671 or the IEE Wiring Regulations. This does not mean that they will fail to achieve conformity with the relevant parts of the Electricity at Work Regulations 1989.*

This is a very important statement by the HSE, demonstrating the importance of BS 7671 in terms of providing compliance with the relevant parts of the Electricity at Work Regulations 1989.

Assessment of medical locations 3

In order to assess the location to provide the correct equipment it is necessary to understand the definitions relating to the categorisation. BS 7671:2008+A3:2015 categorises medical locations into three Groups (0, 1 and 2).

Group 0: medical location where no applied parts are intended to be used and where discontinuity (failure) of the supply cannot cause danger to life.

Group 1: medical location where discontinuity (failure) of the supply does not represent a threat to the safety of the patient and applied parts are intended to be used:

* externally
* invasively to any part of the body except where Group 2 applies.

Group 2: medical location where applied parts are intended to be used, and where discontinuity (failure) of the supply can cause danger to life, in applications such as:

* intra-cardiac procedures; and
* vital treatments and surgical operations.

In determining the classification and Group number of a medical location, it is necessary to involve the relevant medical/clinical staff to identify which medical procedures will take place within the patient environment.

Guidance for the designer is provided by a list of typical medical locations and associated measures, which are indicated in Annex A710 of BS 7671:2008+A3(2015). However, as the list is not exhaustive, in order to correctly determine the classification of a location it is essential to understand:

(a) if ME equipment is intended to be connected to a patient;
(b) if there can be contact between a patient and other persons touching parts of the ME equipment/system; and
(c) whether failure of the mains supply has a detrimental effect on the medical procedure or patient's well-being.

3.1 Understanding the medical procedures

When determining a medical location group rating, it is extremely important for the person carrying out the assessment (usually the designer) to understand what processes and procedures will be carried out in the room or area. It is unlikely that any one person can fully determine all areas without a degree of consultation. Whilst this Guide does not expect the individual engineer to be an expert in procedures, or in anatomy, it is necessary for the engineer carrying out the assessment to have some idea or at least seek out information relating to what goes on in the patient environment.

Correctly assessing a medical location relies on liaison between medical/clinical staff and the electrical engineering designer, who between them are able to discuss the requirements and limitations of the equipment and intended use to arrive at the correct categorization (grouping) of a room or location.

The correct categorization is essential as it may affect patient safety or, if over specified, affect project budgets, which may make the scheme unaffordable or restrict the number of schemes that can be delivered. Both affect patients, one directly, the other indirectly in terms of service availability, so the importance of correct specification and liaison cannot be emphasised enough.

3.2 Determining the group rating

Usually, the categorization of a room or location will be carried out by persons experienced in this process. However, just because you have 'assessed one before' does not mean that you got it right last time!

Using a logical approach to categorization, the following steps are recommended for an individual location or department where there is a client specification and room data sheets:

(a) review the different types of activities declared in the client output specification or the intended activities on the Activity Data Base (ADB) sheet published by the Department of Health or the room data sheet.

(b) check whether the contract documentation relates to any special requirements, for example, references to ME equipment requirements, MEIGaN (now withdrawn), or other special client requirements.

> **Note:** Wherever a withdrawn document is referenced, it is useful to follow up the reason why the document has been referenced. This follow up may reveal that it is a case of poor specification detail or there is a perfectly valid reason. Ultimately, checking details such as this will avoid later confusion.

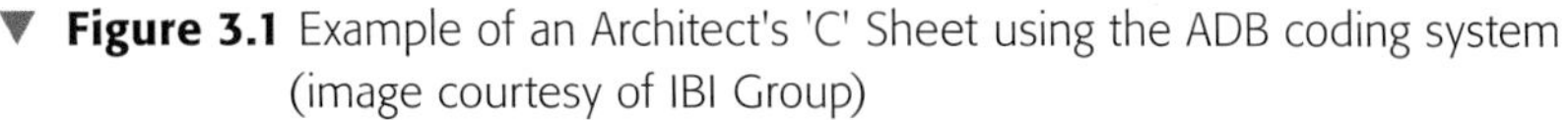

▼ **Figure 3.1** Example of an Architect's 'C' Sheet using the ADB coding system (image courtesy of IBI Group)

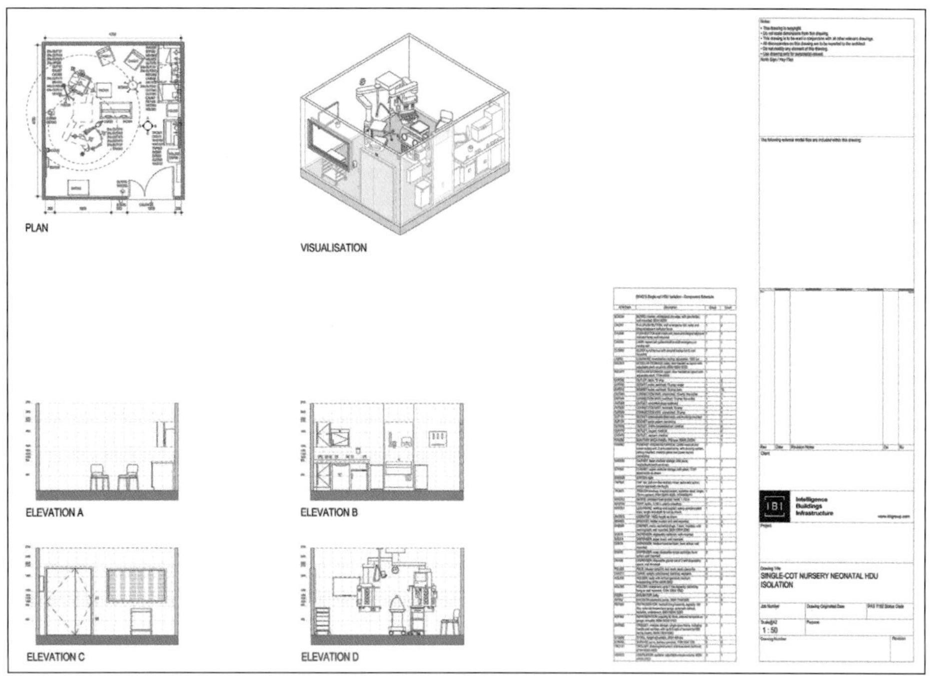

Table 3.1 is an extract of Informative Table A710 from BS 7671. Similar tables are contained in other documents, which are often just rule of thumb guides.

▼ **Table 3.1** Extract from Table A710 from BS 7671:2008+A3:2015

Medical location	Group			Classification	
	0	1	2	≤ 0.5 s	> 0.5 s ≤ 15 s
1 Massage room	X	X			X
2 Bedrooms		X			X
3 Delivery room		X		X[a]	X
4 ECG, EEG, EHG room		X			X
5 Endoscopic room		X[b]		X	X[b]
6 Examination or treatment room		X		X	X
7 Urology room		X[b]		X	X[b]
8 Radiological diagnostic and therapy room		X	X	X	X
9 Hydrotherapy room		X			X
10 Physiotherapy room		X			X
11 Anaesthetic area			X	X[a]	X
12 Operating theatre			X	X[a]	X
13 Operating preparation room			X	X[a]	X
14 Operating plaster room			X	X[a]	X
15 Operating recovery room			X	X[a]	X
16 Heart catheterization room			X	X[a]	X

17 Intensive care room			X	Xa	X
18 Angiographic examination room			X	Xa	X
19 Haemodialysis room		X			X
20 Magnetic resonance imaging (MRI) room		X	X	X	X
21 Nuclear medicine		X			X
22 Premature baby room			X	Xa	X
23 Intermediate Care Unit (IMCU)			X	X	X

a Luminaires and life-support medical electrical equipment which needs power supply within 0.5 s or less.
b Not being an operating theatre.

The 23 medical locations in the above table do not cover all possible medical locations and therefore an amount of interpretation is required.

It is important to define the medical location early in a project so that sufficient space allocation can be made for equipment that may be required, such as distribution boards (DBs), uninterruptable power supplies (UPS) and/or medical IT systems.

3.3 Over-specification

There is a school of thought that believes there is no such thing as over-specification, as it is better to over-provide than to under-provide. That thinking, in the context of the provision of sockets or even number of circuits, may be acceptable for normal situations but over-specification in terms of incorrect medical location classification is a much bigger problem.

Over-specification will cause the project to require additional measures, for example, the inclusion of additional equipment such as a UPS, and maybe even a medical IT system, to meet the strict criteria of a Group 2 location. This equipment will incur additional cost, not only in terms of wiring, equipment and accessories, but also additional spatial requirements, which, in terms of the overall construction budget, will have a profound effect on the project.

A hypothetical example of over-specification, such as specifying a Group 1 location as a Group 2, may add as much as £80k (indicative figure only) of electrical equipment to a scheme. This may be overshadowed by the £200k (indicative figure only) additional construction and structural modifications to take the size and weight of that additional equipment.

Going beyond direct cost, it may be so constraining on space that the scheme is affected in other ways, making the project difficult to deliver.

Such an oversight could be responsible for reducing the overall service provision commissioned or intended, as the healthcare provider can now no longer afford the number of beds or quantity of services required.

Additionally, there are many examples where an attempt to achieve above and beyond the minimum requirements set out in the particular guidance or standard, such as BS 7671, BS 5839 etc., where the designer believes that, by providing an over-provision, they have made an improvement. This belief is a naive approach to design, which should be challenged as over-specification or over-provision is not necessarily the panacea to all design problems; in fact, it can be counter-productive.

Example: over-specification

Taking the example of a designer who decides that all final power circuits in a particular Group 2 location will be supplied by a medical IT system, i.e. all equipment is connected to the medical IT system.

This can be seen by the designer as being an 'improvement' to the requirements as they have given first fault resilience to all electrical equipment in the area. However, this is not necessarily of benefit to the building owner/occupier.

First of all, not all the equipment used in a medical location is actually classified as medical equipment. This might include computers and printers along with other equipment being used in an area. A simplified example of this may be a touch-down area or work station at the end of a resuscitation bed or number of beds, which could theoretically be included in the patient environment; this is more prevalent where the bed position isn't fixed.

As ME equipment is designed and tested to a more stringent standard, which means that there is likely to be less earth leakage on a medical device than a regular piece of equipment with a similar loading. This means that with additional 'ordinary' equipment there is an increased likelihood of the insulation monitoring device (IMD) operating due to the collection of earth leakage currents supplied through the IT transformer.

As medical IT system transformers are limited to a maximum size of 10 kVA for single-phase units, placing all loads on this type of circuit causes unnecessary burdening of IT supplies. Essentially, a greater number of medical IT system final circuits will be required. Also, it is probable that more medical IT transformers will be required, to further supply the department as loadings increase. As the load on the medical IT system increases, the UPS, with its one-hour autonomy is then raised to meet the increased demand.

This increase creates the requirement for a larger battery room to accommodate the load and, as a result of this increase in equipment size, the cooling load has to be increased. In terms of construction, the plant room size has grown along with the structural support for the batteries giving a non-electrical cost increase to the project.

In addition to the increase in size and rating of the plant and equipment, there is a potential for the additional burden to 'destabilise' the alarm and monitoring system due to the amount of normal equipment connected.

A secondary 'side effect' of this design decision is that the very circuits that were intended to be secure and safe to use are compromised by adding unnecessary load from other equipment. It should be noted that adding more load to the medical IT system increases the risk of failure of the IT supply. Ordinary equipment is not designed to the same rigorous standards as ME equipment which could give rise to a potential increase in false or unnecessary alarms on the IT system, which in itself will cause disruption to the clinical service provision.

In addition to the potential for alarm activation through a drop in insulation resistance/leakage currents, the fact that the IT system is being loaded will create additional heat emissions from the medical IT system components. Although the IT cabinets are equipped with ventilation fans, the dissipation of heat from these units can become a burden due to the size of the load added.

Regardless of the effectiveness of the ventilation system within the medical IT cabinet, there is potential for temperature rise within the enclosure. This temperature rise can be attributed to heat not being removed or dissipating from the vicinity (i.e. in a riser or cupboard) or through poor installation practices where the unit does not operate the way it was intended, thus causing a temperature rise inside the unit.

Research into circuit-breaker loadings and behaviours, with respect to ambient temperature and physical location, reveals that standard circuit-breakers have to be de-rated due to temperature and/or whether they are adjacent to each other. There are additional factors that affect the circuit-breaker ratings and that designers should consider when selecting any distribution equipment such as ambient temperature and grouping of protective devices; information relating to this can be found in Appendix 7.

3.4 Under-specification

The consequence of under-specification is slightly more obvious than that of over-specification. However, in many cases under-specification can unintentionally be compensated for by staff and the ME equipment that is used, which can make the under-specification difficult to detect. In these instances it is likely that the design and/or the installation will require modification so that it is brought up to standard some considerable time after the installation has been brought into service.

3.5 Specifications where the client does not require all elements

There are instances where the client does not need or cannot afford all the 'elements' that have been identified for a particular type of medical location. Examples of this may include veterinary surgeons, who, despite using equipment and procedures that are defined as Group 2, are reluctant to provide more measures than a Group 0 or at best a Group 1 location.

In this or similar instances a pragmatic view should be taken. One tried and tested method would be to liaise with the client/clinician to determine exactly what procedures are carried out. Once the ideal classification has been established the client is told what the ideal group rating measures would provide.

Once agreement has been made on the location Group rating of a room or location which would be recorded using an appropriate identification methodology, further discussion with the client is required to discuss safety measures should be provided so as to make the installation no less safe than if full compliance were to be in place. This would involve looking in detail into the mitigation gained by each measure applied to the electrical design. Where this cannot be achieved then a separate client control measure will need to be put in place. Each control measure should be reasonable with a process in place to ensure the measure does not fail.

An overall assessment should then be documented so that the resulting arrangement allows the client to provide an environment that is no less safe than if compliance with the regulations or requirements had been achieved.

This is a risk-management approach to determining the medical location; it is not a risk-taking exercise or a money-saving measure to be applied in every instance/ project. This approach is not dissimilar to the intended departure requirements set out in Regulation 120.3 or the new materials and inventions requirements of Regulation 133.5 of BS 7671.

For example, for a high street veterinary surgeon, the requirement for access to alternative supplies, generator back-up plus tertiary supplies with a medical IT system giving first-fault protection may seem a little 'over the top'. There is often little opportunity to provide alternative supplies and a generator to provide the basic infrastructure. As there is little evidence of death by failure in electrical systems in animals, it will be difficult to persuade a veterinary surgeon that they need lots of specialist installation equipment, beyond the specialist ME equipment that will be used as part of the procedure being performed.

Consequently, despite a medical location being typically Group 2, it is likely that there will be a considerable gap between the measures that are required and those that the client is prepared to accept. The designer in conjunction with the client, who in this scenario is deemed to understand the clinical risks, should document and record the process and considerations that have been made which result in the final design and installation. The resulting document will provide evidence demonstrating that all parties are aware of the relevant risks and consequences of not applying certain requirements. It will also indicate what mitigation measures have been put in place to remove any danger. Where the measures cannot achieve a required level of mitigation then the original requirements should be applied or the installation would be considered non-compliant.

Despite this apparent flexibility in approach, this Guide supports the theories developed in line with international standards. It promotes the use of designs that have assessed the relevant risks, which in turn provides a level of assurance, demonstrating all design decisions are fully considered. Information supporting this consideration should be detailed in risk assessments/design statements that should be provided with the design and included in the operation and maintenance information for future use/reference.

A Guide to Electrical Installations in Medical Locations
© The Institution of Engineering and Technology

Risk assessment 4

In order to bridge the gap between the requirements of Section 710 and the client-perceived requirements, a risk assessment/design statement should be put into place. This should leave all parties clear as to how each risk identified has been mitigated where possible, where a risk cannot be mitigated and what measures, that are aligned with BS 7671, have been introduced to make the installation acceptable.

▼ **Figure 4.1** Risk assessment/design statement

MEDICAL LOCATION ASSESSMENT/DESIGN STATEMENT								
Client Name			Project Name Address		Measures Agreed Y/N	Design Initials	Clinical Initials	Director Initials
A710 Rating	Room description: Detailed description of room use	Compliant	Comments		Agreed Rating			
Reg No/ Clause No	Description of regulation	Y/N	Comments including clinical reasons		Measures Agreed Y/N	Designer Signature/Initials	Clinicians Signature/Initials	Director Signature/Initials
	Detail of departure or requirement		Mitigation details					

POST CONSTRUCTION ASSESSMENT							
Reg No/ Clause No	Description of regulation	Y/N	Comments including clinical reasons				
	Detail of departure or requirement		Mitigation details/implemented				
Review Date:	Review observations/actions Any significant changes since design agreed?						

The use of this document is an iterative process and should be carried out as soon as possible in the design briefing stage, and then again as the design develops. This risk assessment should also be included in the final design in the form of a design statement.

During the final construction period, it is recommended that this information, including design decisions etc., be included in the final verification information, such as the operation and maintenance manuals, with a link to the documentation in the original Electrical Installation Certificate along with sufficient information for those carrying out maintenance and future inspection reporting.

A simple risk assessment is shown in Appendix 5.

4.1   Variations to BS 7671

There is a culture within healthcare construction to derogate against particular technical guidance documents, which is recorded in a derogation schedule. It is important to remember that BS 7671 cannot be derogated against.

BS 7671 is configured so that compliance is also likely to meet the requirements of the EAWR. Where absolute compliance cannot be achieved due to a new invention or process that was not available at the time of publication of BS 7671, this is dealt with by the designer who will need to declare an intended departure, in accordance with Regulation 120.3 or, for new materials and inventions, Regulation 133.5. This intended departure is then declared on the Electrical Installation Certificate in conjunction with any relevant risk assessment/design statement relating to the intended departure. The intended departure should have been considered by the designer and the resulting degree of safety of the installation should not be less than that obtained by compliance with the Regulations.

Whilst this approach may not be an ideal one, it is a practical and pragmatic approach to manage both clinical and engineering challenges, where the standard requirements may not deal with the specific issues.

The risk assessment format indicated above has been used in live projects. However, it is not simply applied without considerable thought. The assessment is used to review different risks and apply additional measures appropriate to the procedures and interventions taking place in a particular location, with the net result being that a system design is no less safe than a system applying Section 710 to a 'normal' or foreseen circumstance.

A point worth noting is that, whilst most locations are similar, the designer should never underestimate the possibility that the clinical procedures in one room will be different in another, even within one department.

As a cautionary word it is useful to remember that no one is right all the time; we are after all only human. A term often heard when challenging an existing approach is "we have done this on the last four new hospital projects", to which I often reply, "does that make it right or is it that you have made a number of unchallenged mistakes?"

Repeating a process because it was done last time or in a similar room may seem to make commercial sense, however, this practice risks the introduction of multiple errors or even out-of-date practice.

4.2   Common understanding

There should always be adequate liaison with all parties so that everyone's needs are understood. A tick-box approach may be contractually satisfactory but will fall significantly short of the mark in achieving an optimal design.

A simple example of poor understanding is easily explained in clean utility lighting control design using presence detection, where the brief to the designer states that "the lights go on and off as you use the room, helping to meet energy targets and Approved Document L compliance" (for England and Wales). The end user is pleased as their lights will work when they want them to and go off when not in use.

The situation is not as ideal as might be expected: often, clean utility is used to store drugs and, in certain instances, sharps are used. One such example is that of a nurse who is stood still counting controlled drugs, or carrying out fine motor movements. A considerable amount of time might have lapsed before there is any movement detected by the lighting sensor, plunging the nurse into darkness whilst holding or 'drawing up' medicines with a sharp needle, or losing count of a number of controlled drugs, which have to be accounted for – or worse, losing concentration whilst preparing or administering medicines. Whilst it is possible to simply extend the time delay, the whole point of presence detection may then be lost.

In terms of the message that is being delivered it is essential both parties need to understand what is being offered and what is being accepted. The designer didn't tell any untruths but forgot to ask what activities were carried out in the room. If the designer fully understood the activities in the room they may not have suggested that type of switching.

Equally, if the end user knew or had been told that the lights went out when the occupants were stationary, they too would not have accepted the lighting control as proposed.

Once installed it is either difficult or expensive to rectify, which then results in a compromise to avoid significant costs. This would typically be to adjust the relevant timers so that the room will have lights that stay on for twenty minutes. This excessive overrun will be necessary to prevent the lights being switched off creating a hazard on a very infrequent basis. Consequently, the energy saving is potentially lost as the lights are then often hardly ever off especially if the room is often used throughout the day, even for a matter of seconds.

This compromise can make the lighting control for the room ineffective and possibly counter-productive in terms of energy saving.

Errors such as this are normally removed by having a common understanding for all parties with a policy of 'there is no such thing as a stupid question' approach in place. This allows for a proper explanation, which in the above scenario would have eradicated this very trivial error and a more appropriate solution found at the briefing/ design stage.

A Guide to Electrical Installations in Medical Locations
© The Institution of Engineering and Technology

Review of existing locations 5

As BS 7671 is not retrospective, there is therefore no direct requirement to upgrade an installation each time there is a change made to that standard – as doing so would be unnecessary and impossible to maintain.

However, even though BS 7671 is not retrospective, there is a requirement for those who own and maintain the estate to ensure that what is installed is both functional and does not present a danger to users and those maintaining it. The following process will be necessary for owner-occupier's estate managers and consultants tasked with carrying out an appraisal of existing infrastructure. A level of skilled judgement needs to be applied, as it is unlikely that a one-fit solution exists in the medical location due to the varying factors, which could include review of:

(a) the age of the existing installation;
(b) the types of procedures carried out;
(c) how the existing system is supported by safety power supplies etc.; and
(d) the impact of the unaltered system to stakeholders.

It is therefore necessary to review each medical location on its particular merits and restrictions. Following an inspection or review of an existing location it may be necessary to carry out some consequential improvement works. This may be due to the fact that the procedures carried out in this area are far in excess of those intended at the point of original design or that clinical techniques have moved on requiring additional power requirements.

In existing installations, particularly where an installation is aged, every alteration or amendment intended to be carried out should be preceded with a full analysis of risk to ensure that the intended work is appropriate. The assessment should also make sure that the modifications have not made the installation less resilient and hence affecting safety as a consequence of meeting a particular requirement.

An example of this would be the application of RCD protection to final circuits: where there is only one lighting or power circuit to a large area, the loss of circuit through the operation of an RCD could have disastrous consequences. In this instance by not going far enough with the alterations, such as restructuring the final circuit arrangements to minimise outage and leave other circuits intact e.g. providing additional lighting or power circuits to an area in order to minimise the impact of a final circuit failure could render the electrical installation more at risk to failure. Hence it is important to consider any modification works and the impact that applying limited consequential improvement to an installation. For example, in Section 710 RCD lighting is required but, to minimise the impact of an RCD trip, multiple lighting circuits are required. This, therefore, addresses the additional protection against electric shock balanced with the impact of local circuit failure.

5.1 Common causes of confusion when assessing a medical location

Most, if not all, healthcare-related construction contracts have a requirement to comply with the HTM or SHTM series of documents, and they must also meet the requirements of BS 7671. This 'dual' compliance needs to be understood by the relevant parties. At the time of publication, HTM 06-01A(2007) in particular is out of synch with the current edition of BS 7671, with references to BS 7671:2001 throughout (SHTM 06-01A being published later has more up-to-date, but not current, references). A common cause of misinterpreting a medical locations group rating occurs by the way the risk is categorised in HTM 06-01 and the designer trying to apply this directly to Section 710.

Although I personally advocate the reading and assessing of risk profiles contained in HTM 06-01 (Part A), it is important that the information obtained does not confuse or distract the designer from the assessment process required by Section 710 of BS 7671. It is therefore important to note that a medical location assessment according to BS 7671 assesses the location primarily on the basis of risk to the patient predominantly through discontinuity (failure) of supply, whereas the wider requirements of a healthcare facility, such as a hospital, have more far reaching implications, including, but not limited to, high voltage systems (which are outside the scope of BS 7671).

The HTM and SHTM series of documents include matters beyond the immediate requirement for resilient or back-up supplies as they address the wider impact of clinical service delivery, for example, the surgeon cannot operate successfully if the cleaner hasn't cleaned the theatre. These matters are important and represent a separate but very important facility for the business continuity element and medical support services.

HTM 06-01A is currently not maintained to the same refresh cycle as BS 7671; however, at the time of publication an update is under way with modification to SHTM 06-01 2011 under consideration.

5.2   HTM 06-01 risk profiling

A great deal of confusion can exist for persons trying to categorise various locations as they search through existing documents, practices, understandings and misunderstandings within the industry. The first principle to understand is that the systems presented within BS 7671 and HTM 06-01 are not directly compatible with each other. This is more than likely due to both timing of publications and the way the two documents have been developed. In many instances they produce similar results although in some areas different results are produced depending on how the documents are interpreted and supplied.

Most professionals will be familiar with the risk profile arrangements set out in HTM 06-01A:2007, in which the document sub-divides risk into two categories: clinical risk and non-clinical risk.

Clinical risk is further subdivided into patient and non-patient areas: patient clinical risk, and non-clinical and business continuity risk.

▼ **Figure 5.1** Patient clinical risk category (from HTM 06-01(2007) courtesy of the Department of Health (DoH))

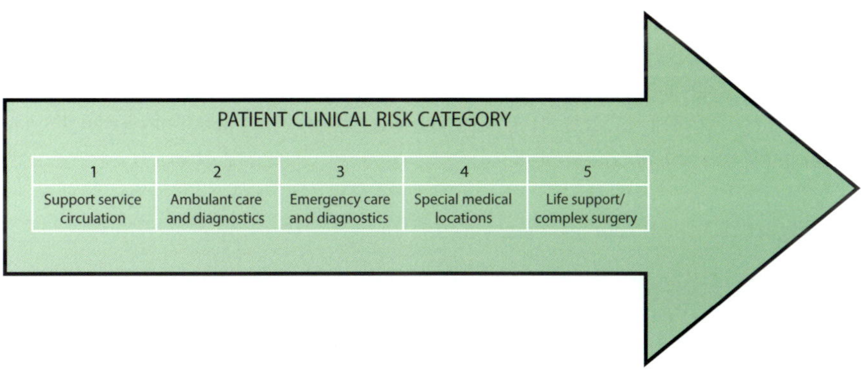

Non-clinical risk is subdivided into medical and engineering services.

▼ **Figure 5.2** Non-clinical and business continuity risk category (from HTM 06-01(2007) courtesy of the DoH)

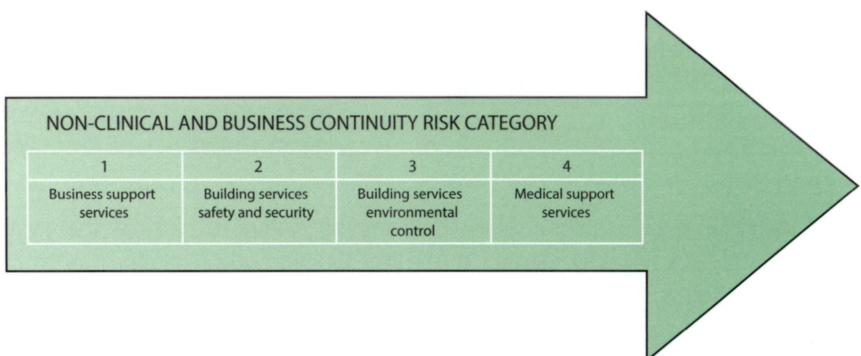

In trying to apply logic to these subdivisions, which are based on pre-2007 health models of care, HTM 06-01 acknowledges that there is no rule that definitively places healthcare premises in any one category or defines one category for a particular healthcare site, particularly for small healthcare premises such as GP practices and health clinics or centres.

HTM 06-01(2007) states that Risk Category 1 and 2 areas are deemed not to relate directly to IET Guidance Note 7.

Adding to the confusion, Risk Category 3 includes mention of mental health wards and some maternity units, which, although possibly appropriately applied to Risk Category 3, could easily fall into a higher category.

The confusion is compounded as the HTM does identify performance requirements in Risk Category 3 areas, suggesting that both medical gases and access to a standby power system is required. However, the basis for the classification of all locations should be determined by what medical procedures are carried out, rather than by a departmental name, ward type or premise size.

As the clinical risk category increases, the alignment with Section 710 improves, as there is considerable parity between the higher clinical risk categories and the requirements of Section 710 of BS 7671.

As previously identified, many designers are faced with the difficulty of being contracted to meet the (S)HTM and BS 7671 requirements simultaneously. Currently, both documents have different approaches to certain elements. The responsible designer should look to comply with BS 7671 but, where the standard is silent on a matter or detail, the guidance in HTM or SHTM should then be applied.

Despite referencing IEC 60364-7-710, which was current at the time of drafting, HTM 06-01(2007) takes its own approach, which also includes the HV infrastructure (HV is outside the scope of BS 7671). Risk profiling in HTM 06-01 is meant to be applied to distribution strategies, which are assessed in a table of electrical failure risks, evaluated to clinical categories.

▼ **Figure 5.3** Distribution strategy (from HTM 06-01, courtesy of the DoH)

RISK OF ELECTRICAL FAILURE BY INFRASTRUCTURE

Risk by clinical category (refer to Chapter 4 under 'Clinical risk')	Distribution strategy (refer to Chapter 6)				
	Primary supply: unified distribution (Fig.14)	Primary and secondary supply - unified and segregated distribution (Fig. 15)	Primary and secondary supply - unified and dual unified distribution (Fig. 16)	Dual-primary and dual-secondary supply - unified and dual-unified infrastructure (Fig. 17)	Dual primary and dual HV secondary supply - dual unified infrastructure (Fig. 18)
Life support complex surgery	HIGH	HIGH	SIGNIFICANT	MODERATE	LOW
Special medical locations	SIGNIFICANT	SIGNIFICANT	MODERATE	MODERATE	LOW
Emergency care and diagnostic	MODERATE	MODERATE	MODERATE	LOW	RESIDUAL
Ambulant care and diagnostic	MODERATE	MODERATE	LOW	LOW	RESIDUAL
Support services and circulation	LOW	LOW	RESIDUAL	RESIDUAL	RESIDUAL

Although this table is useful when determining a level of risk, as the system was not developed to directly identify a medical location group rating, it is of little help in determining a definite number for the group and, consequently, an element of judgement is still required.

Once a medical location group rating has been determined, the suitability of the infrastructure can be assessed and mitigations put in place by using some of the techniques employed in the HTM risk-profile procedure.

5.3   Assessment of risk: summary

Both systems work independently of each other and, although apparently addressing the same risks, the early attempts to define medical locations by the HTM authors prior to the international standards being incorporated into BS 7671 have left a mismatch between the two systems, particularly in some of the lower classification areas.

Regardless of the above, it has to be recognised that HTM 06-01A in 2007 (and subsequently SHTM 06-01A in 2011) took a major step forward in taking a risk-management approach to installation design and decision making. However, the conservative approach of having to spell out what is and isn't a particular risk or hazard has meant that there are subtle differences between the HTM risk assessment process and the categorisation of medical locations in BS 7671.

It should be remembered that when categorising a location, there is a level of irrelevance to the name of a room or who provides the service. Instead, it is about the procedure, application of applied parts and the risk to life should there be a fault or discontinuity of the electrical supply to equipment in that location.

If and when a designer is faced with a challenge between complying with the specific (S)HTM requirements or those of BS 7671 then the following simple rule should be applied:

Refer and design to BS 7671; where the standard and its supporting guidance is silent, refer to the HTM for assistance. The information in the HTMs is for guidance and should not contradict the requirements of BS 7671.

In making any assessment of a location or when looking at a complete building/facility, the overall service delivery element will need to be considered to assess the wider impact of medical locations. Consequently, to simply class a full hospital solely in terms of the Group 0, 1, 2 definitions would be insufficient as wider service delivery is equally important.

Where the designer varies from either of these documents, BS 7671 or (S)HTMs, they should ensure that the solution is no less safe than if full compliance were to be achieved.

A Guide to Electrical Installations in Medical Locations
© The Institution of Engineering and Technology

Risks to patients: shock {#6}

Shock hazards due to bodily contact with the 50 Hz mains supply are detailed in IEC/TR2 60479-1 *Effects of current on human beings and livestock – General aspects.* The IEC 60479 suite of documents deals with contact with electricity in non-medical conditions and cannot therefore be reliably used for guidance in medical locations.

▼ **Figure 6.1** The diagram from IEC/TR 60479-1 with associated interpretation

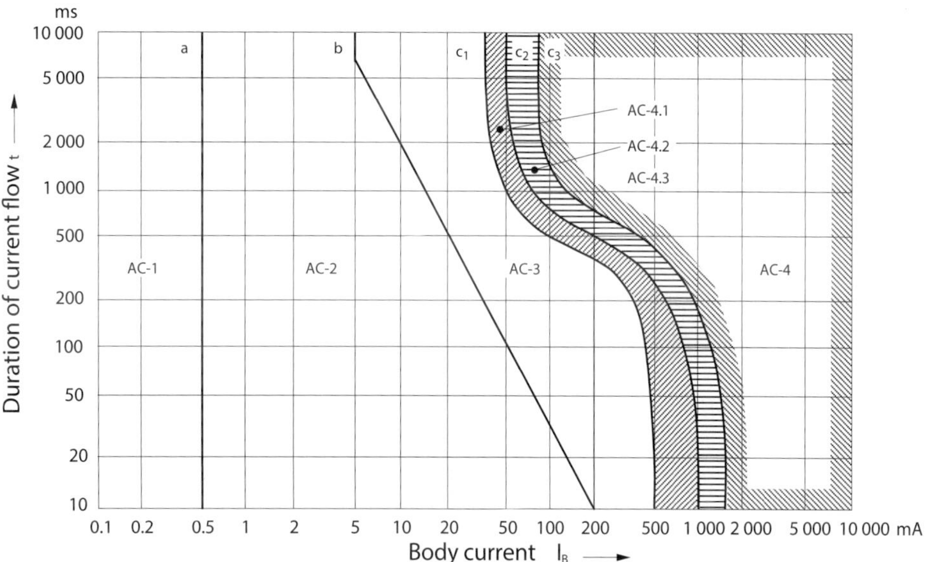

▼ **Table 6.1** The effects of current on the human body (Table 4 of IEC 479-1)

Zone designation	Zone limits	Physiological effects
AC-1	Up to 0.5 mA (curve a)	Perception possible but usually no 'startled' reaction
AC-2	0.5 mA up to curve b	Perception and involuntary muscular contractions likely but usually no harmful electrical physiological effects
AC-3	Curve b and above	Strong involuntary muscular contractions. Difficulty in breathing. Reversible disturbances of heart function. Immobilisation may occur. Effects ncreasing with current magnitude. Usually no organic damage to be expected

Zone designation	Zone limits	Physiological effects
AC-4	Above curve c1	Patho-physiological effects may occur such as cardiac arrest, breathing arrest, and burns or other cellular damage. Probability of ventricular fibrillation increasing with current magnitude and time
AC-4.1	Between c1 and c2	Probability of ventricular fibrillation increasing up to about 5 %
AC-4.2	Between c2 and c3	Probability of ventricular fibrillation up to about 50 %
AC-4.3	Beyond curve c3	Probability of ventricular fibrillation above 50 %

Note: For durations of current flow below 200 ms, ventricular fibrillation is only initiated within the vulnerable period if the relevant thresholds are surpassed. As regards ventricular fibrillation, Figure 6.1 relates to the effects of current which flows in the path left hand to feet. For other current paths, the heart current factor has to be considered.

The standard chart from IEC/TR 60479-1 and the table from IET Guidance Note 5 *Protection Against Shock* does not take into account that the natural protection of the human body is considerably reduced when certain clinical procedures are being performed on it. Patients under treatment may have their skin resistance broken or their defensive capacity either reduced by medication or nullified while anaesthetised. These conditions leave the patient vulnerable to the effects of electric shock.

HTM 06-01A deals with both clinical and business risk. When it comes to clinical risk, stringent measures are necessary to ensure the safety of patients in medical locations. These measures are required where patients are undergoing procedures where the loss of mains supply may pose a risk to safety and where there is an increased risk from shock under fault conditions.

6.1 Development of appropriate thresholds

Research indicates that currents of the order of 10 mA passing through the human body can result in muscular paralysis followed by respiratory paralysis depending on skin resistance, type of contact, environmental conditions and duration. Eventual ventricular fibrillation can occur at currents just exceeding 20 mA. These values are quoted in both HTM and Guidance Note 7.

In patient environments where intra-cardiac procedures are undertaken, the electrical safety requirements for medical equipment are more strict than in other locations in order to protect the patient against 'microshock'. Patient leakage currents from applied parts introduced directly to the heart can interfere with cardiac function at current levels that would be considered safe under other circumstances.

Existing guidance indicates that the patient leakage current that can flow into an earthed patient is normally greatest when the equipment earth is disconnected. Limits are set as to the amount of leakage current that can flow in the patient circuit when the protective earth conductor is connected (normal condition) and disconnected (single fault condition). Patient leakage currents of the order of 10 µA have a probability of 0.2 % for causing ventricular fibrillation (VF) when applied through a small area of the heart. In the same conditions with a leakage current of 50 µA, which is considered a microshock, the probability of ventricular fibrillation, according to BS EN 60601-1, increases to 1 %. The values quoted have often been misinterpreted, leading to significant confusion regarding safety in electrical installations in medical locations.

BS 7671 does not deal with ME equipment as it is outside its scope. It is important to remember that most, if not all, interventions use ME equipment of some description. As a designer, installer or maintainer of ME installations it would be remiss to ignore the equipment and the vital role it plays in patient safety.

The information provided in this Guide does not challenge the work identified in IEC/TR 60479-1 and previous electrical guidance, but instead recognises the use of ME equipment in procedures.

6.2 Leakage current: background

All mains-powered electrical equipment will have some degree of leakage current, which must be kept within safe limits to prevent any electric shock hazard. These leakage currents arise from capacitive, inductive or resistive coupling between the mains parts and the enclosure or other conductive parts of the appliance. Since there is no such thing as a perfect insulator, all electrical devices will have some degree of leakage current.

In all appliances there are two types of leakage currents that can normally be measured:

(i) protective conductor leakage current, which is sometimes referred to as equipment earth leakage current; and
(ii) touch leakage current, which is sometimes referred to as enclosure leakage current.

Due to the use of applied parts of ME equipment that are directly connected to a patient, there are additional leakage current measurements that need to be taken. These additional leakage currents are:

(i) applied parts leakage current;
(ii) F-type applied parts leakage currents; and
(iii) applied parts patient auxiliary current.

One point to note is that, for both medical and non-medical appliances, the leakage currents measured will be worse when either the earth or the neutral conductor is in an open circuit. The reason for this is demonstrated by Figure 6.2.

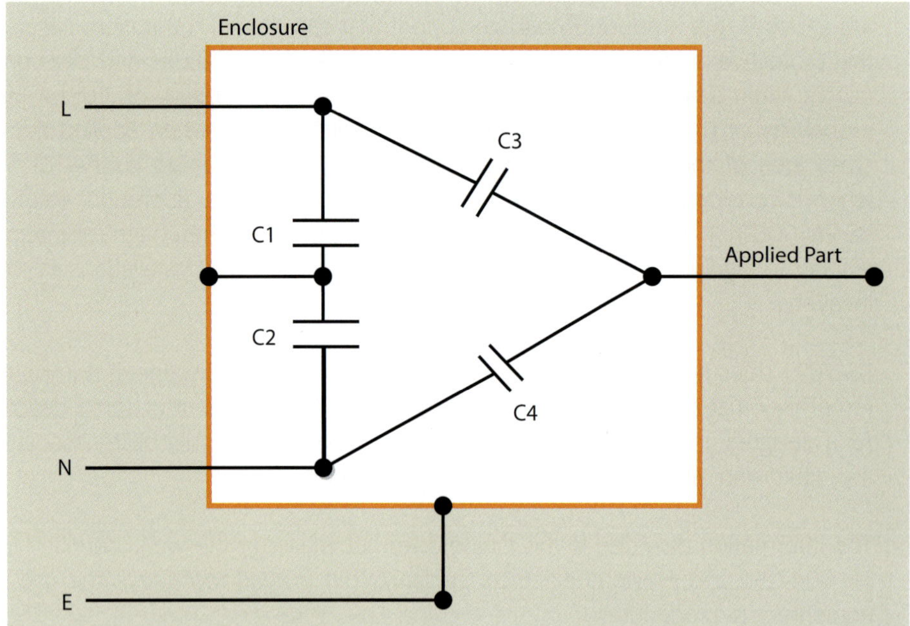

▼ **Figure 6.2** Simplified diagram of an appliance

Since, in most modern appliances, the leakage current consists mainly of capacitive elements, the diagram focuses on these. C1 and C2 represent the capacitive coupling from the supply to the enclosure. In fact, these are often actual capacitors found in many appliances to reduce radio frequency interference (RFI) and to comply with electromagnetic compatibility (EMC) requirements. C3 and C4 represent the capacitive coupling between the mains part and any secondary parts of the equipment. These can be applied parts, as shown in Figure 6.2, or equally could be conductive parts of the appliance that are isolated from earth, such as a metal handle or accessible conductive parts of a Class II appliance.

▼ **Figure 6.3** Normal condition

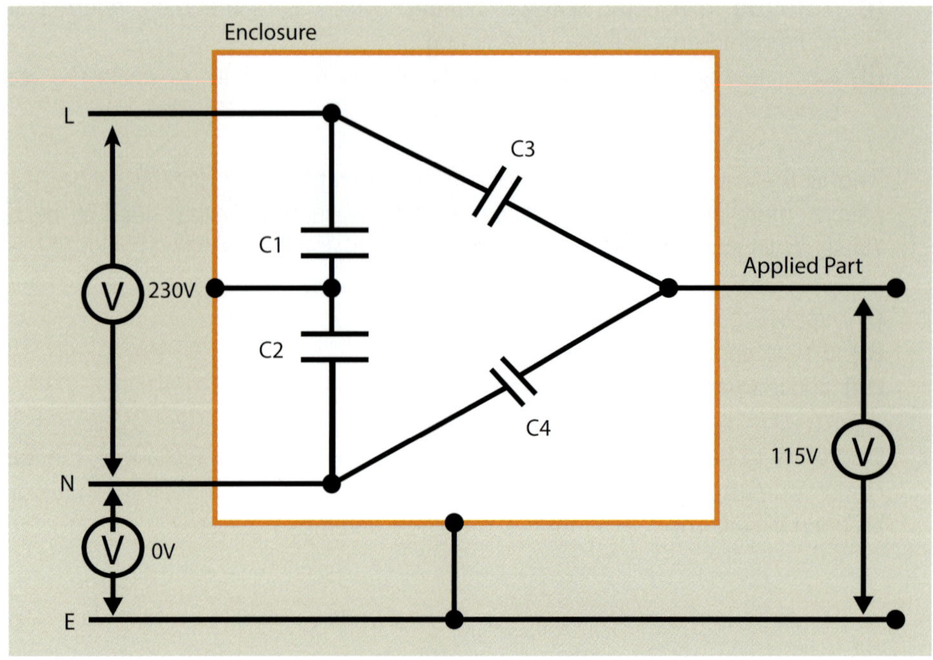

The leakage current flowing into the appliance earth connection is, in normal conditions, made of the current flowing through C1. If the live and neutral are transposed then the primary leakage will be due to C2, which is why it is important to make measurements with both polarities in CENELEC countries other than the UK. The leakage current to the applied part connection is made up of the current that flows through C3, attenuated by the current that flows in C4. Since, when loaded by the impedance of the human body, the voltage across C4 is almost zero, the primary leakage current is solely due to C3.

If we use a high impedance voltmeter we could expect, in normal conditions, to measure the voltages shown in Figure 6.3. The 115 V measure on the applied parts connection is due to the potential divider made up of C3 and C4, since it is quite normal for the capacitance values of this coupling to be equal. Clearly, when loaded by the normal resistance of a human body (1,000 Ω for medical locations and 2,000 Ω for non-medical locations) this voltage will drop to a very low, safe value (about 0.1 V for a Type B applied part).

▼ **Figure 6.4** Single fault condition

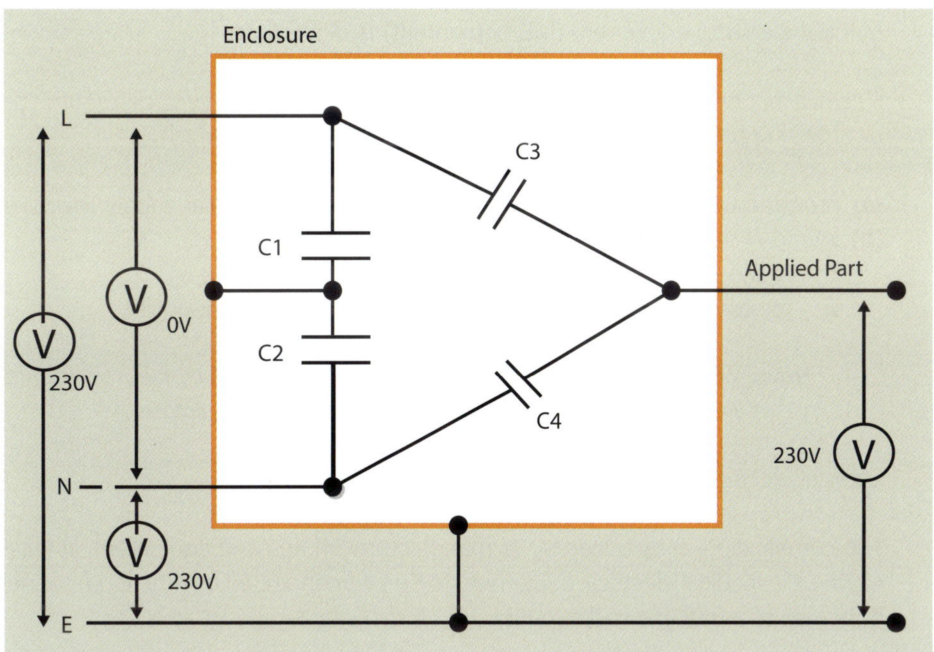

Figure 6.4 demonstrates what can happen under single fault conditions (SFC) where the neutral becomes open circuit. The leakage current flowing into the appliance earth connection is made up of the current flowing through C1 and C2, as they both have the full supply voltage across them. This leads to the possible doubling of the measured leakage, assuming C1 and C2 are equal. Also, since C3 and C4 now have the full mains supply presented, the leakage measured for the applied parts connection will naturally increase.

The full voltage of the mains supply is present on both C3 and C4 and the voltage on the applied parts connection, measured with a high impedance meter, has risen to the full mains potential of 230 V. Again, this would still rapidly collapse to a safe voltage once loaded by the resistance of a human body (about 0.5 V for a Type B applied part).

This should explain why two limit values are set for appliance leakage current values: one for normal conditions and one for fault conditions.

It should also be evident that making measurements with a high impedance voltmeter, which most meters are these days, may lead to possibly alarming values being measured, unless you understand the nature of their origin.

6.3 Normal equipment example

It is possible to perceive the small difference in potential between Class II equipment and sensitive parts of the body, such as the back of the hand, when in contact with true Earth.

This is evident even on a laptop chassis. Even though a laptop may be supplied by a Class II (double insulated) power supply, it is possible, with a high impedance voltmeter, to measure up to half the mains supply voltage between the accessible conductive parts and earth. This Guide does not advocate trying this out in case of damage to equipment.

6.4 Medical electrical equipment (ME equipment)

Medical electrical equipment (ME equipment) is defined as:

Electrical equipment having an applied part or transferring energy to or from the patient or detecting such energy transfer to or from the patient and which is:

(a) provided with not more than one connection to a particular supply mains; and
(b) intended by its manufacturer to be used:
    i   in the diagnosis, treatment or monitoring of a patient; or
    ii   for compensation or alleviation of disease, injury or disability.

> **Note:** ME equipment includes those accessories as defined by the manufacturer that are necessary to enable the normal use of the ME equipment.

Medical electrical system (ME system) is defined as:

The combination, as specified by its manufacturer, of items of equipment, at least one of which is medical electrical equipment to be interconnected by functional connection or by use of a multiple socket-outlet.

> **Note:** the system includes those accessories that are needed for operating the system and are specified by the manufacturer.

All ME equipment must meet the requirements of the Medical Device Directive (93/42/EEC). In the UK these are the Medical Devices Regulations and they are issued under the Consumer Protection Act 1987.

Since EU regulations apply directly to the UK they do not need to be transposed. The most common method of ensuring compliance with the directive requirements is by using equipment that conforms to IEC/BS EN 60601 series of documents.

ME equipment is rigorously tested and maintained to meet the performance requirements of BS EN 60601 and the Medical Device Directive.

The earth-connected state is referred to as 'normal condition' (NC) and the disconnected earth is referred to as 'single fault condition' (SFC). Limits are set for the protective conductor leakage, enclosure or touch leakage in addition to the leakage currents for any patient connections, which are known as applied parts.

Different types of ME equipment in use can be generally categorised, for the purpose of medical locations, by the type of applied parts (parts that are in contact with the patient) that they use. The three main types of applied parts are B, BF and CF as defined in BS EN 60601, and are shown in Figure 6.5 along with the allowable leakage current limits. The level of touch leakage is set by the categories defined in BS EN 60601-1.

▼ **Figure 6.5** Types of applied parts

Symbol	Applied part type	Definition/description	Normal Condition (NC)	Single Fault Condition (SFC)
	Type B Applied Part	**TYPE B APPLIED PART** APPLIED PART complying with the specified requirements of BS EN 60601 to provide protection against electric shock, particularly regarding allowable PATIENT LEAKAGE CURRENT and PATIENT AUXILIARY CURRENT	100µA	500µA
	Type BF Applied Part	**TYPE BF APPLIED PART** F-TYPE APPLIED PART complying with the specified requirements of BS EN 60601 to provide a higher degree of protection against electric shock than that provided by TYPE B APPLIED PARTS	100µA	500µA
	Type CF Applied Part	**TYPE CF APPLIED PART** F-TYPE APPLIED PART complying with the specified requirements BS EN 60601 to provide a higher degree of protection against electric shock than that provided by TYPE BF APPLIED PARTS	10µA	50µA

The above values are for a.c. current and for a single applied part only. Other values exist for d.c. and multiple applied parts.

There are other sub-categories defined in BS EN 60601, however, they relate to specifics, such as defibrillator-proof versions of these three main types of applied parts.

Notes:
- A sub-section of any standard can override the main standard, so, for example, X-ray units are allowed a higher earth leakage than is normally allowed by the main standard.
- The touch leakage current limit (such as touching the equipment chassis, handle or other accessible parts) is set at the same level as B-type applied parts.
- F-type parts (BF and CF as defined by BS EN 60601) are always isolated from earth and must be able to withstand the application of 250 V AC applied between them and earth.
- B-type parts may be connected to a protective earth or isolated from earth.

6.5 Types of applied parts

The selection and use of ME equipment is outside of the scope of this Guide but the complex safety requirements of ME equipment and the patient environment are very important.

Referring back to the significant classifications in BS EN 60601, the applied parts are described as follows:

> TYPE B APPLIED PART
>
> TYPE B APPLIED PARTS provide the lowest degree of PATIENT protection of all the types of APPLIED PART and are not suitable for DIRECT CARDIAC APPLICATION.
>
> The PATIENT CONNECTION(S) of a TYPE B APPLIED PART could be:
>
> – PROTECTIVELY EARTHED;
>
> – connected to earth but not PROTECTIVELY EARTHED; or
>
> – floating, but not isolated from earth to the degree that would be required for a TYPE BF APPLIED PART.

Type B applied parts typically consist of:

- operating table;
- X-Ray table or chest stand; and
- weighing scales.

> TYPE BF APPLIED PART
>
> TYPE BF APPLIED PARTS provide a degree of PATIENT protection higher than provided by TYPE B APPLIED PARTS. This is achieved by isolating the PATIENT CONNECTIONS from earthed parts and other ACCESSIBLE PARTS of the ME EQUIPMENT, thus limiting the magnitude of current that would flow through the PATIENT in the event that an unintended voltage originating from an external source is connected to the PATIENT, and thereby applied between the PATIENT CONNECTIONS and earth. However, TYPE BF APPLIED PARTS are not suitable for DIRECT CARDIAC APPLICATION.

Type BF applied parts typically consist of:

- defibrillator;
- blood oxygen monitor;
- ultrasound machine; and
- ECG machine.

> TYPE CF APPLIED PART
>
> TYPE CF APPLIED PARTS provide the highest degree of PATIENT protection. This is achieved by increased isolation of the PATIENT CONNECTION from earthed parts and other ACCESSIBLE PARTS of the ME EQUIPMENT, further limiting the magnitude of possible current flow through the PATIENT.
>
> TYPE CF APPLIED PARTS are suitable for DIRECT CARDIAC APPLICATION insofar as PATIENT LEAKAGE CURRENT is concerned, though they could be unsuitable in other respects, such as sterility or biocompatibility.

Type CF applied parts typically consist of:

- ECG machine;
- contrast injector; and
- intra-cardiac ultrasound machine.

Reviewing the above examples, it is obvious that the same type of equipment is seen in more than one category of applied parts. (It should be noted that it is possible for a single piece of ME equipment to have multiple applied parts within the same device.) This is due to the type of procedures being performed, which can be varied. For example, an ultrasound machine used for scanning a knee only needs to be BF but an ultrasound machine used to scan inside the vessels of the heart must be CF rated. Using the wrong machine for the procedure being performed could be very dangerous.

The three main categories of applied parts are set out so that, for particular interventions, the equipment is constructed so that maximum protection is given to the patient for the type of intervention or procedure being carried out.

6.6   Protective conductor current

Protective conductor current can be present either as part of a fault or due to the 'leakage' of a device under normal conditions. 'Earth leakage' current depends on mains voltage, capacitive and inductive coupling along with any other resistances to earth.

In Figure 6.6, an example is indicated in the Class I piece of equipment, which has a leakage current of 10 mA flowing with a 230 V supply, equating to an approximate impedance of 23,000 Ω. The person touching the casing should be free from harm, as this current is safely flowing through the equipment earth connection.

▼ **Figure 6.6** Class I equipment

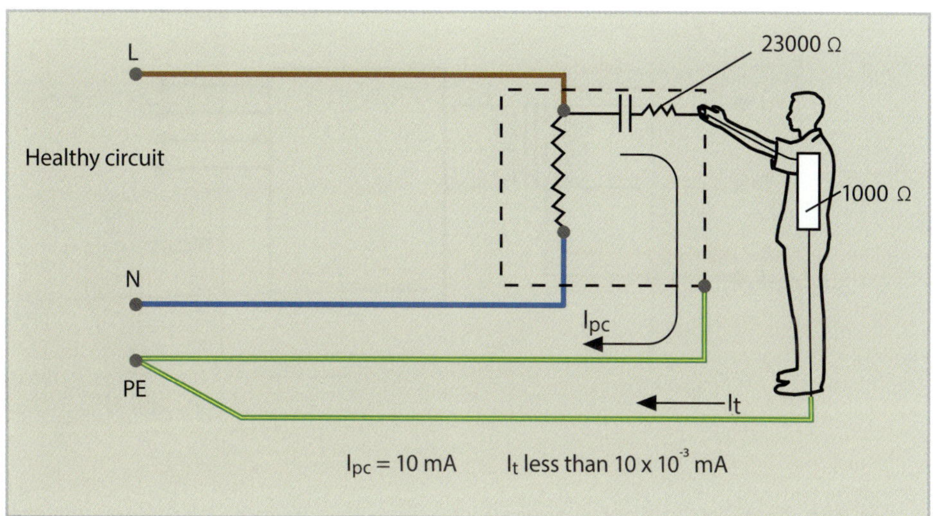

Within a medical location the average resistance of the human body is assumed to be 1,000 Ω. Outside of a medical environment it is assumed to be 2,000 Ω.

Should there be discontinuity of the protective conductor, the person touching the casing is likely to become part of the circuit. Applying the impedance of the leakage in series with the body's impedance gives a total of 24,000 Ω, with a corresponding current flowing of 9.6 mA. This is demonstrated in Figure 6.7.

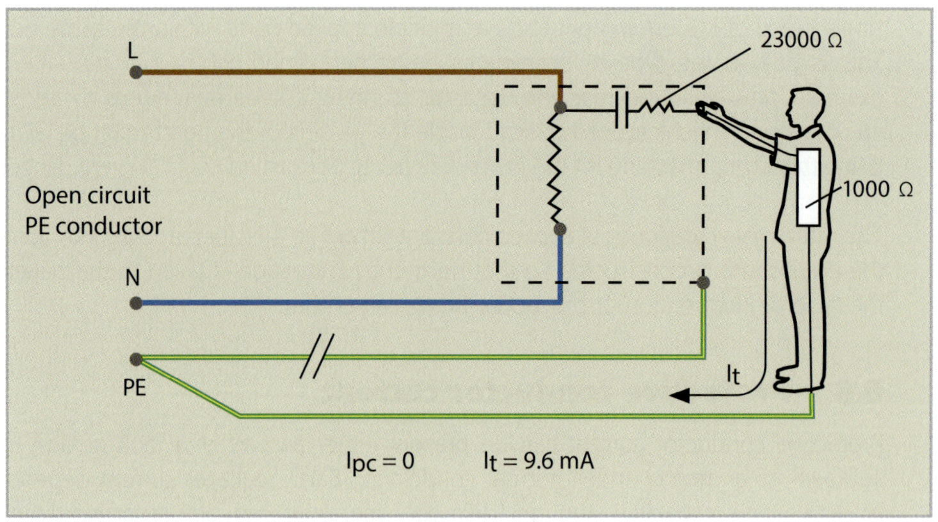

▼ **Figure 6.7** Protective conductor current flow

6.6.1 Earth leakage current

In ME equipment, a protective conductor current can flow in Class 1 equipment as indicated in Figure 6.8.

▼ **Figure 6.8** Protective conductor current flowing in Class 1 equipment

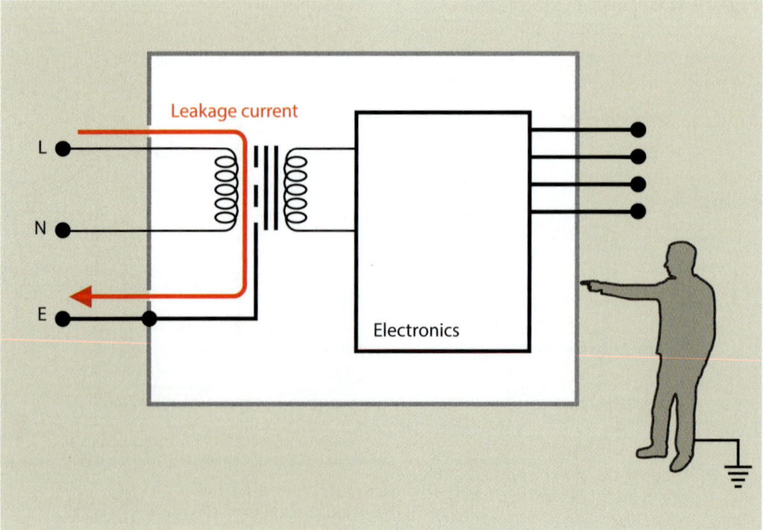

As with any piece of Class 1 equipment, where the equipment is adequately earthed the patient and operator should not be at risk under first fault to earth condition. Due to the more stringent requirements in medical locations, equipment complying with the Medical Devices Directive or BS EN 60601 must be within predetermined strict limits, which in turn satisfy patient safety requirements.

6.6.2 Touch leakage current

Touch leakage current is also known as enclosure leakage current. Touch leakage current is the current that flows from the enclosure to earth, excluding patient connections, through a conductor but not a protective conductor. This can be current induced into conductive parts not connected to earth, which would equate to touching Class II equipment. The limit is 100 µA in normal conditions and 500 µA in single fault conditions, such as an open circuit earth or an open circuit neutral.

▼ **Figure 6.9** Touch leakage current

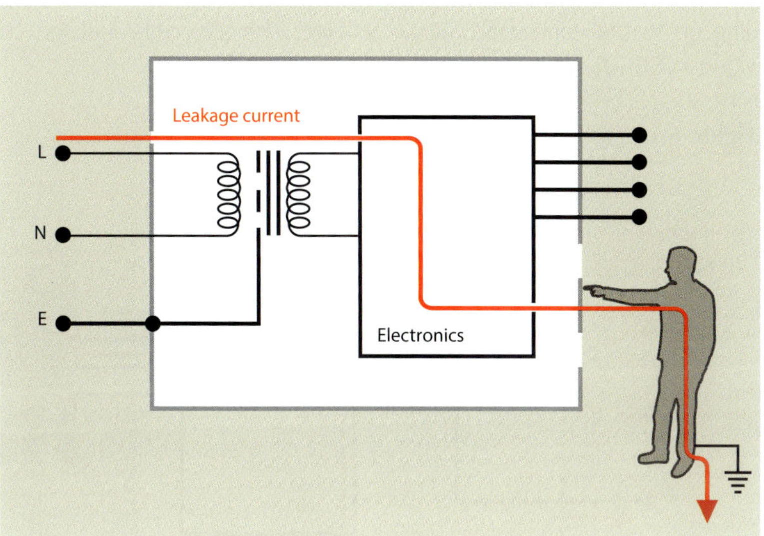

6.6.3 Patient leakage current

Patient leakage current is the current that flows through the applied part(s) to earth via a patient. An example of this would be current that flows via electrocardiogram (ECG) machine connections. The values of patient leakage current are measured in both normal and single fault conditions (a single fault may be an open earth or neutral).

BS EN 60601 determines the maximum allowable current for a particular type of applied part, for example, B, BF or CF.

▼ **Figure 6.10** Patient leakage current

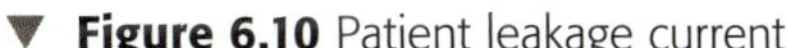
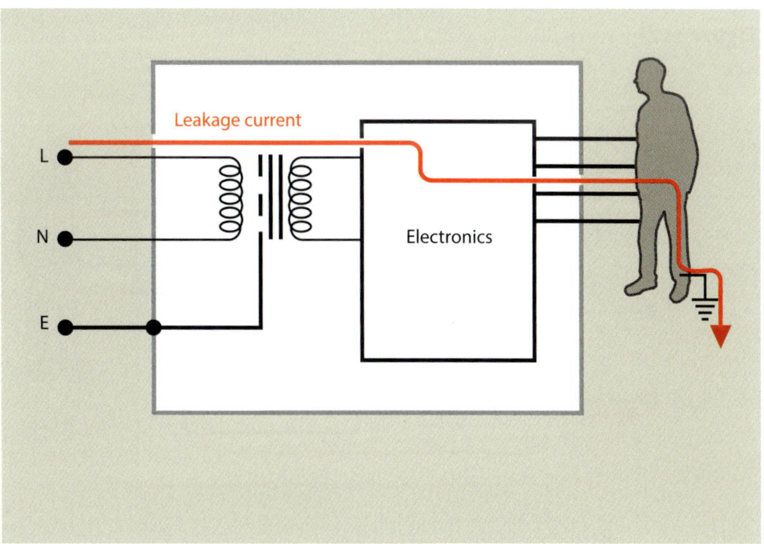

6.6.4   Patient leakage current F-type parts only

In F-type applied parts patient leakage current can flow from an external source, via the patient and the applied parts, to earth. This is sometimes known as mains-on applied parts. Examples of these F-type parts include ultrasound probes and ECG electrodes. Either could be BF or CF, depending on the clinical application.

An example of where this voltage may come from is when a Class II device secondary or unearthed electrical item comes into contact with the patient; it can also originate from the applied parts of other ME equipment. It should be noted that when presented with a high impedance load, any leakage currents will result in a measured voltage reading up to the connected supply voltage. The allowable leakage current limit is provided in 60601-1.

▼ **Figure 6.11** Patient leakage current F-type parts only

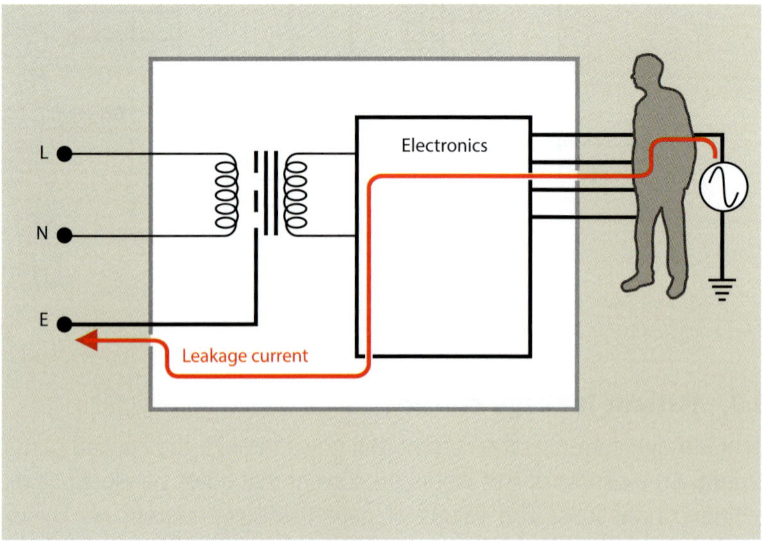

6.6.5   Patient auxiliary current path

Patient auxiliary current path is the current that flows between parts of the applied part through the patient and that is not intended to produce a physiological effect. This is predetermined at product design stage and is only ever of interest to the persons who may be designing new medical devices.

▼ **Figure 6.12** Patient auxiliary path current

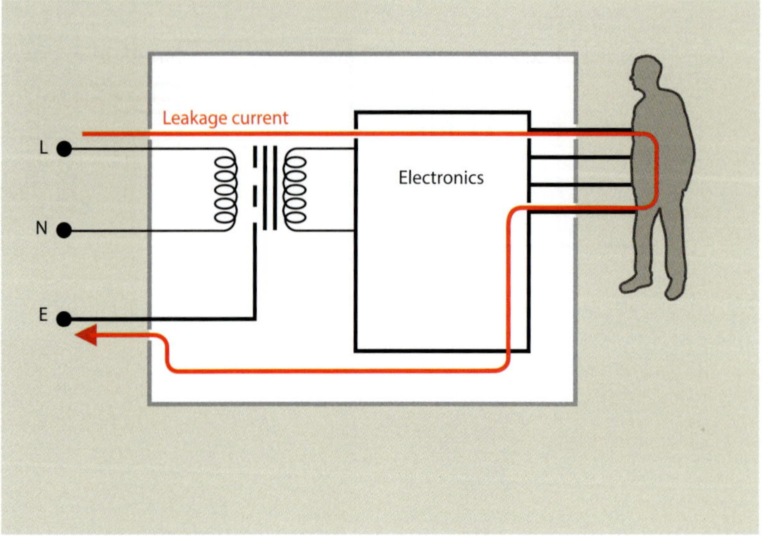

6.7　Equipment type: summary

It can be shown that:

(a) the natural protection of the human body against electric shock is considerably reduced when certain clinical procedures are being performed on it;
(b) the natural protection of the skin resistance is reduced when it is cut or broken;
(c) the defensive capacity of the patient is either reduced by medication or nullified while anaesthetised; and
(d) very small currents (μA) can interfere with the heart's pumping action.

Previous approaches to medical location design have tended to look at the medical location to meet performance requirements for heart catheterisation and similar processes, which mentioned maximum currents of 10 μA and 50 μA (sometimes referred to as 10 mV and 50 mV touch voltages).

Whilst this Guide does not challenge the values of leakage currents, it has to be recognised that medical procedures that take place rely on a number of factors, including:

(a) medical and clinical staff;
(b) processes and procedures adopted by clinical staff during medical investigations;
(c) medical equipment/ME equipment/medical electrical systems; and
(d) medical location electrical installation.

The staff, processes and procedures are key to ensuring patient safety, as is the selection and correct use of ME equipment. For example, improper handling of catheters while inserted into the heart may lead to dangerous conditions caused by mechanical or electrical stimulation. Touch current could conceivably reach an intra-cardiac site if careless procedures are used when handling intra-cardiac conductors or fluid-filled catheters. Normal clinical practice would ensure that such devices are always handled with great care. This is also reflected in BS EN 60601-1, which rates the probability of direct contact between an intra-cardiac device and the ME equipment enclosure (earth) as only 1 in 100 medical procedures.

It should also be clear that the electrical installation couldn't be considered a medical device, as it would be impossible to ensure it conformed to all the requirements of the medical device directive or BS EN 60601-1. Although many previous publications have mentioned the need to limit touch voltages or leakage currents to specific levels, as though it were a medical device, in practice this would be impossible to design for in advance. Some previous publications have tried to assume that the installation protective earth could contact the heart and so have set limits in line with CF applied parts. Clearly, the electrical installation should never contact the heart directly, as only medical devices, which conform to strict requirements, are allowed to make this sort of electrical connection. Although inadvertent contact via the medical staff has a 1 in 10 probability, applying the strict requirements of BS 7671 Section 710 ensures that excessive touch currents are highly unlikely to occur.

Further information is supplied in Appendix 4 Supplementary information.

The patient environment may seem to be straightforward in terms of the dimensions given in Figure 7.1, however, the bed location is not always fixed and the wider patient area should be assessed.

▼ **Figure 7.1** Patient environment – from Figure 710.1 in BS 7671

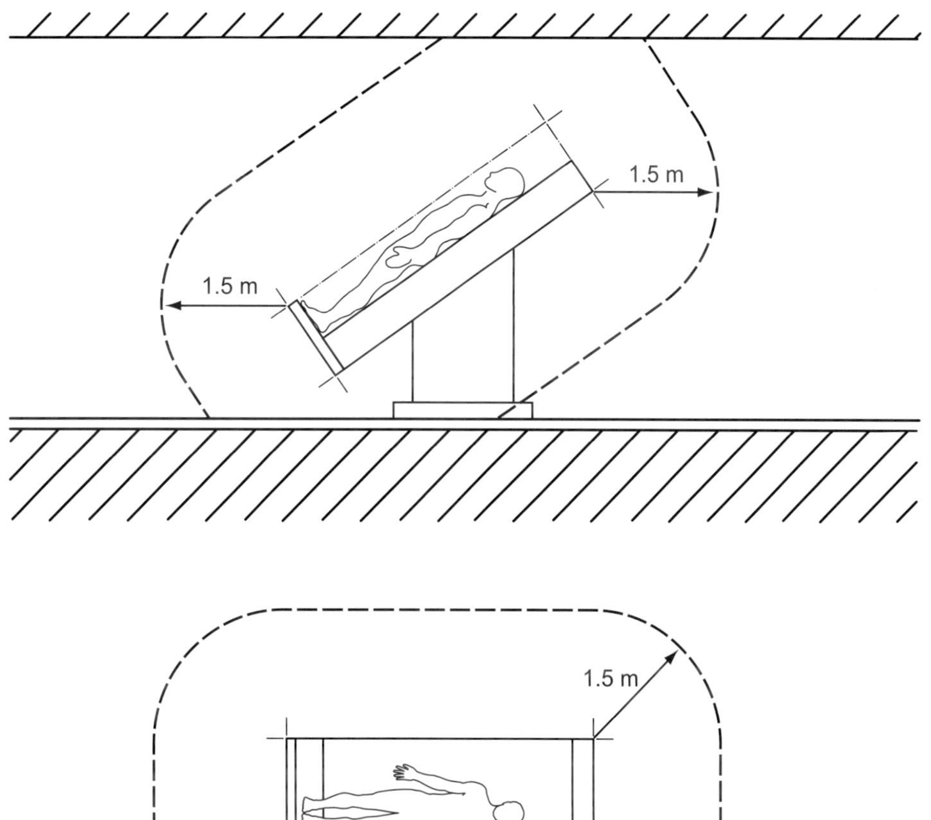

The arrangement above applies when the patient's position is pre-determined; if this is not the case, all possible patient positions should be considered in the location. It is possible to find that the patient environment is not fixed and therefore covers a greater area than may be first thought. In the first instance the bed position is relatively firm.

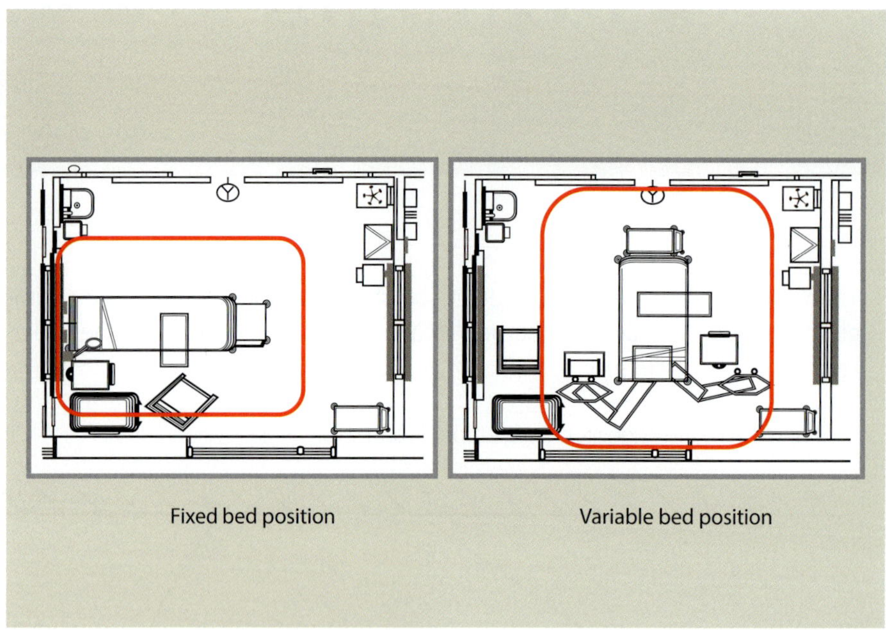

▼ **Figure 7.2** Patient environment with fixed and variable bed positions

The above example contains two identical sized rooms on the same project; the first has wall-mounted fixed medical gases and medical services in a wall-mounted arrangement, the second has articulated medical pendants. As can be seen, the patient environment is much larger due to the variable bed location.

The impact of the larger patient environment affects the area in which supplementary equipotential bonding is required. This is particularly important on retrofit and upgrading schemes. On new projects the requirement does not significantly affect the design as the current trends are towards the provision of large amounts of supplementary equipotential bonding. However, on site it is important that local supplementary equipotential bonding is carried out properly to ensure that Regulation 710.415.2 is met. In meeting this regulation, the impedance of any bonding is such that the voltage present between simultaneously accessible exposed-conductive-parts and/or extraneous-conductive-parts does not exceed 25 V AC or 60 V DC in accordance with Regulation 710.411.3.2.5.

During an inspection of a site that I had been involved in the design of, I came across a document called 'Earthing Record' that the site electricians had created. Although it was very much based on their earlier works using MEIGaN, they had applied it to a Section 710 installation. There are other examples that cover more than just supplementary equipotential bonding, examples of which are included in the appendices of this Guide.

▼ **Figure 7.3** Supplementary Equipotential Bonding record

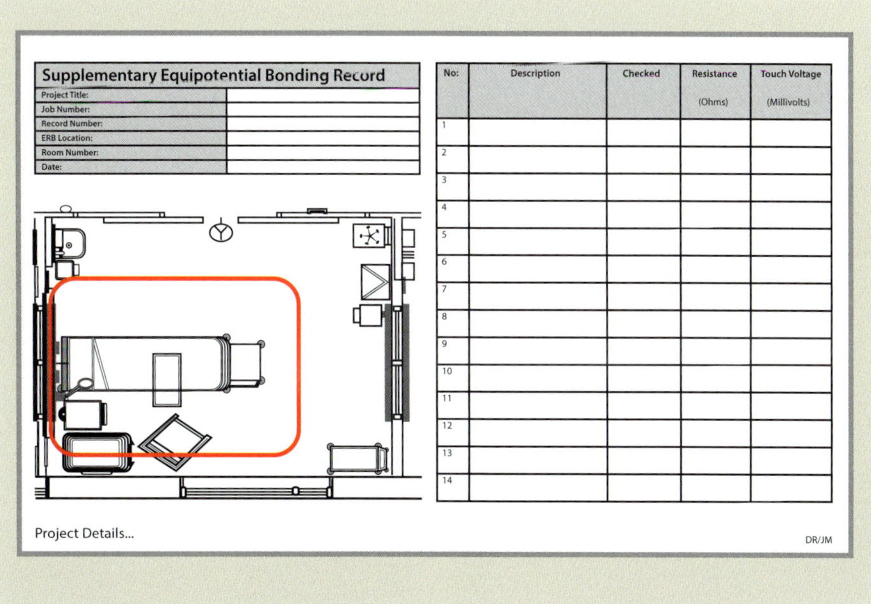

The 'Earthing Record', which has been retitled 'Supplementary Equipotential record', had been produced to ensure that, during the works, the correct conductors had been incorporated and, importantly, had identified the full extent of the patient environment.

This document is able to be used as part of the commissioning process and ultimately forms part of the Operation and Maintenance (O&M) record information and design statement information.

It records the details, impedance and the reference of the Equipotential Bonding Busbar (EBB), room reference etc. Although preparing this document involves some of the rigorous processes reminiscent of the now withdrawn MEIGaN document, this type of information is invaluable in providing very important initial test information and future O&M information so that the periodic inspection requirements relating to periodic inspection can be achieved.

Medical locations have additional requirements above and beyond those of the risk from electric shock. Some electrical equipment (life-support equipment, surgical equipment, etc.) perform such vital functions that loss of supply would pose an unacceptable risk to patients. In such locations, supplies are governed by specific requirements related to their reliability, availability and resilience.

8.1   Resilience

The dictionary meaning of resilience is 'generally to be able to withstand adverse events'.

The fundamentals of resilience can be applied in varying degrees to any system. The level of resilience will usually be dictated by the need for the electrical systems to withstand adverse events. These events may include loss of supply, or cable fault or similar.

Resilience of the electrical installation within a building or complex that supplies any location can be improved by examining what I see as the four Rs:

(a) Reliability of equipment and ability to change components on failure;
(b) Reparability (ability to repair or replace components on failure);
(c) Redundancy; and
(d) Removal or relocation of a single point of failure.

Reliability: this can be assessed as the mean time to failure (MTTF), i.e. how long a component will last in service or, on average, how long a component or system will remain serviceable.

Reparability (ability to repair or replace components): this is of particular importance in systems that are critical to the business operations of the client. Consequently, easily accessible and readily available components combined with a recognised and safe change-out process is essential. This is often the ability to manually put the system in bypass to replace a faulty component.

Redundancy: this means that there is more than one supply available, i.e. should one supply fail there is a redundant supply available to take up the load. Examples of this would include damage to a supply cable or a total failure in the supply.

A truly redundant public electricity supply is usually not possible to achieve due to the constraints laid down by the Distribution Network Operator (DNO). It falls upon those designing the systems to look at the highest level of reliability they can provide to build a resilient system. The designer has to therefore provide a system of secondary power. This secondary power system should be as reliable as possible, able to meet the load demand placed upon it and be able to supply any safety service connected to the supply. It is usual for these secondary power supplies to meet the requirements of an electrical source for safety set out in BS 7671, which means that the supply and associated equipment will also be subject to the additional requirements set out in Chapter 56 of BS 7671. Load profiles and protection should be configured to ensure a reliable supply for the installation.

8.2 Single point of failure

Single points of failure are points in any system where one failure will cause total disruption of the supply or service provision. For example, with any dual-fed piece of equipment, at some point the redundant supply will need to meet the regular supply and at that point the two supplies are vulnerable. These points in a system cannot be completely removed from the system however, they should be moved as close to the point of use as possible.

Solutions range from separate cable routes or fire resistant cabling/enclosures to selecting the position of any changeover units etc.

▼ **Figure 8.1** Example of supply for two theatres

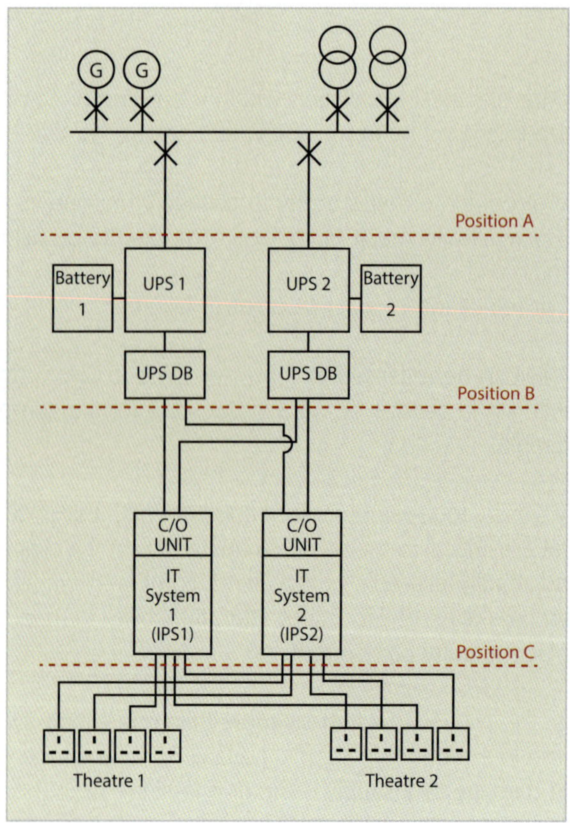

Figure 8.1 indicates a simple but resilient system that would be required for a typical pair of theatres. The medical IT systems would be considered to be in an N+1 arrangement. As BS 7671 requires at least one transformer per room or functional group of rooms, then provided they are considered a functional group by way of clinical use then the N+1 statement is correct. They would also require sufficient UPS and battery autonomy to supply both theatres from any one supply. This arrangement, without a substantial external influence, has sufficient resilience to ensure that a normal component failure or first fault will not significantly affect the supplies.

Hypothetically, by placing a fault at different points along the route, it is possible to find if there is a single point of failure.

In Figure 8.1, despite the low voltage (LV) mains being supported by generators (in case of loss of supply), if a significant fault or the cable route is subjected to fire at, or slightly upstream of, position A, there would be loss of both supplies. HTM 06-01 advocates that there be alternative supplies available, however, if they are all routed through the same corridor or duct there is an obvious single point of failure.

Rectification at Position A: this is achieved by addressing the routing of the supply cables so that they do not share the same route or entry point and are as separate as possible until the last moment of joining. Alternatively, this can be addressed by using fire-resistant cables and putting different cables on different containment routes, creating segregation so far as physical constraints or practicality will allow. Provided that the cabling is PH120, the cables will have a two-hour fire resistance period if the cable has been designed in accordance with BS EN 8519, which allows for cables to operate under fire conditions in accordance with specific requirements.

A similar scenario exists at **Positions B** and **C**. It is unusual to use fire-resistant final-circuit cabling given that a fire in the area will normally render the area unable to be used. However, it may be the case that the medical IT system has been located separately and passes through an area that may be subject to fire, but the end user is in another fire-free area. That end user will still require power even if only to finish a procedure etc. Fire survival is discussed further in Section 9.

8.3 System selection

An assessment of primary and secondary supplies available will need to be performed for all possible configurations of the electrical infrastructure elements taking into account the effects of different technologies. Each will have risk-mitigation strategies associated with the possibility of power failures occurring. The overall risk of power failure occurring can be mitigated by the correct selection of element configurations and interconnections.

In most healthcare sites, the buildings are supplied from their own high voltage to low voltage (HV-LV) transformers, which are 99.999 % available, equating to 5.25 minutes of unavailability per year. Generators, with their moving parts, potential for failures and variables such as load and temperature, have an availability of 99.995 %, equating to 4.5 hours non-availability per year. Simply by adding generators to the electrical supply infrastructure results in the electrical supply availability being increased and, as a result, resilience is improved.

The supply to a medical location needs to be resilient to support both patient safety and business continuity. Both HTM 06-01 and SHTM 06-01 for Scotland set out the required resilience expected from the electrical infrastructure to meet the requirements of clinical risk for a given location or area. They also discuss different types of non-clinical activity, both of which may have very specific requirements.

The clinical risk categories are defined in HTM 06-01:2007 as follows:

(a) Category 1 – support service circulation;
(b) Category 2 – ambulant care and diagnostics;
(c) Category 3 – emergency care and diagnostics;
(d) Category 4 – patients in special medical locations; and
(e) Category 5 – life support or complex surgery.

The clinical risk areas differ from the definitions related to medical locations in Section 710 of BS 7671 and are discussed in Section 5 of this Guide.

> **Note:** The risk categories defined above are to be amended in the updated version of HTM 06-01.

Fire survival 9

Healthcare premises are covered by the requirements set out in the FireCode series of documents, which includes HTM 05-02 *FireCode guidance in support of functional provisions (Fire safety in the design of healthcare premises)* 2015. The requirements of fire survival of the electrical infrastructure are important in healthcare premises as both life support and fire-fighting applications are applicable and are referenced in HTM 05-02.

9.1 Escape is not always the option

In large healthcare premises such as hospitals it is not always feasible for patients to escape from the building when the fire alarm has been activated. In these instances patients and staff, where necessary, avoid or escape any fire and smoke by implementing progressive horizontal evacuation (PHE), which is a procedure to avoid leaving the building. This is to avoid putting patients and any associated medical equipment outside the building and exposed to the elements which may be detrimental to their health and well-being.

▼ **Figure 9.1** Examples of Escape Routes indicated in HTM 05-02 (courtesy of the DoH)

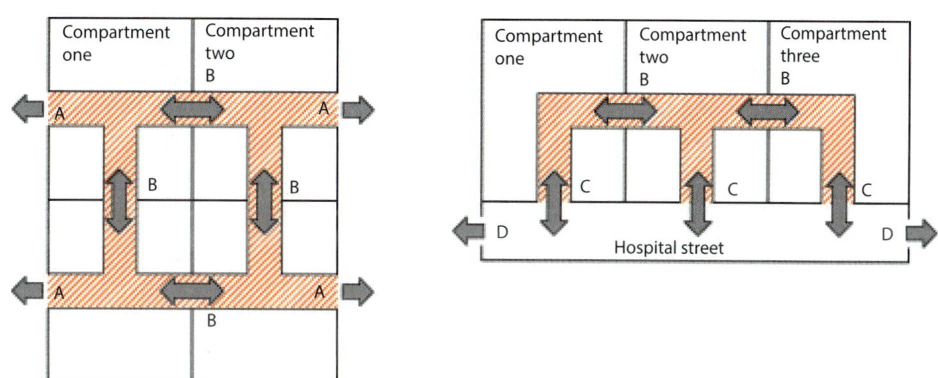

Movement of high dependency patients (such as patents in intensive care, those undergoing surgery and patients in areas which would often be, but are not limited to, locations that are classified as a Group 2 location) is usually a last resort, it is important that the medical equipment providing life support and their associated electrical supplies are available even under onerous conditions such as a fire in an adjacent compartment.

This is in contrast to many other types of buildings where the major concern is for escape and for the fire and rescue services to be able to access and fight the fire.

9.2 Application of fire survival considerations

BS 8519 identifies electrical loads, which are defined as life safety and firefighting loads, and looks at a variety of factors to be considered. One such factor is performance requirements related to fire survival time – the period of time during which the electrical distribution system is maintained with integrity under defined fire conditions.

The requirements of fire survival of the electrical infrastructure is important in healthcare premises as both life support and firefighting applications are applicable and are referenced in BS 8519.

BS 8519:2010 *Selection and installation of fire-resistant power and control cable systems for life safety and fire-fighting applications – Code of practice* was produced in response to the increased height and complexity of buildings as well as the necessity of meeting the fire protection required by both standard arrangements and fire engineered solutions.

It is important to remember that although HTM 06-01 (2007) does not directly reference this ability to be fire resistant, HTM 05-02 does call for electrical distribution systems serving life safety or fire-fighting applications, as detailed in BS 8519, to have resistance to the effects of fire.

Due to the large number of different electrical supply options and variations of medical locations, the number of considerations would be too large to consider in this Guide. However, focusing on Group 2 locations and the medical IT systems required by BS 7671 can give an indication of some of the considerations that should be made; these considerations could then be applied to different supply scenarios.

9.3 Medical IT system supplies

Standard configurations typically depicted by the HTM/SHTMs, the medical IT system, UPS etc. is in the same fire compartment as the area it serves. In this scenario the only real consideration is to try to segregate the supply cables within relevant areas. This can be achieved by using fire segregated construction, e.g. by use of separate risers and diverse routing, which will add to the resilience. However, in many instances large amounts of equipment is often located in remote plantrooms which often creates additional challenges for designers.

Where equipment is located remotely, sometimes the supply cables may have to pass through other fire compartmented areas to serve the 'target' area/location. Where this occurs there is a possibility that a fire could occur in an adjacent fire compartment and, even though the structural fire precautions, dampers etc. operate as planned and the high dependency patient is in 'relative safety', they are then potentially compromised by loss of electrical supply, which may affect lights, power or a combination of both.

With this in mind the designer and installer should consider what I call the 'what if' scenario, which is a process of identifying what would happen if a fire were to occur in an adjacent compartment.

Below are examples of how fire protection of cables to medical IT systems can be considered in slightly different configurations within the same system.

▼ **Figure 9.2** Remote UPS with supplies passing through other fire compartment

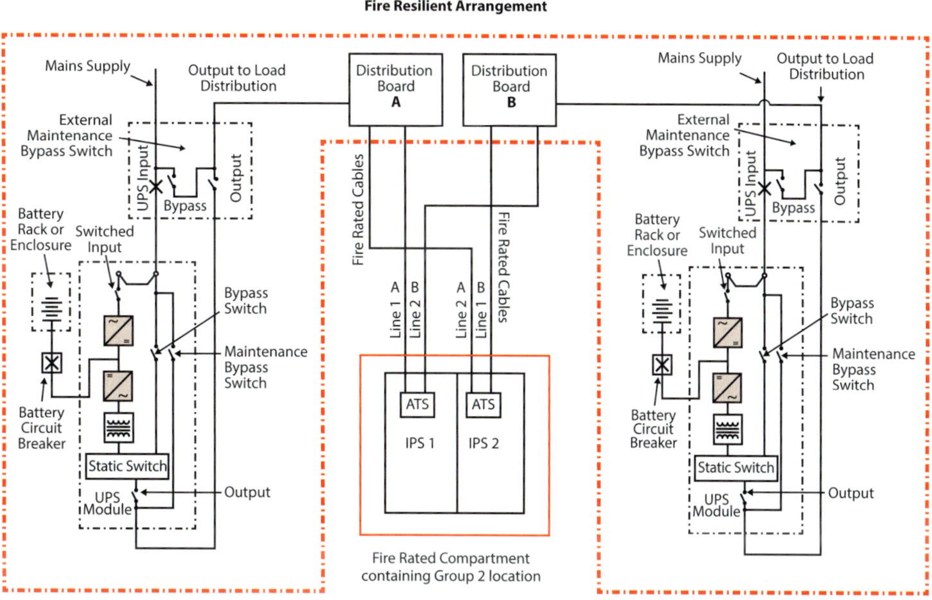

In Figure 9.2, the UPS and the distribution circuit that supply the IT cabinets are in a fire segregated plant area, which may be close to or even on the floor above. However, the medical IT cabinets are located within the same fire rated compartment as the high dependency patient. Consequently, there would be limited benefit in providing fire resistant final circuit cabling as a fire in that compartment would require occupants to move regardless of dependency.

Should a fire occur between the plantroom and the fire rated compartment, without suitable fire protection, the medical IT cabinet supplies may be compromised, resulting ultimately in loss of power to medical equipment.

The effect of providing fire rated cabling mitigates the potential loss of supply to the IT cabinets and ultimately to the medical equipment.

▼ **Figure 9.3** Remote UPS supplies to IT systems

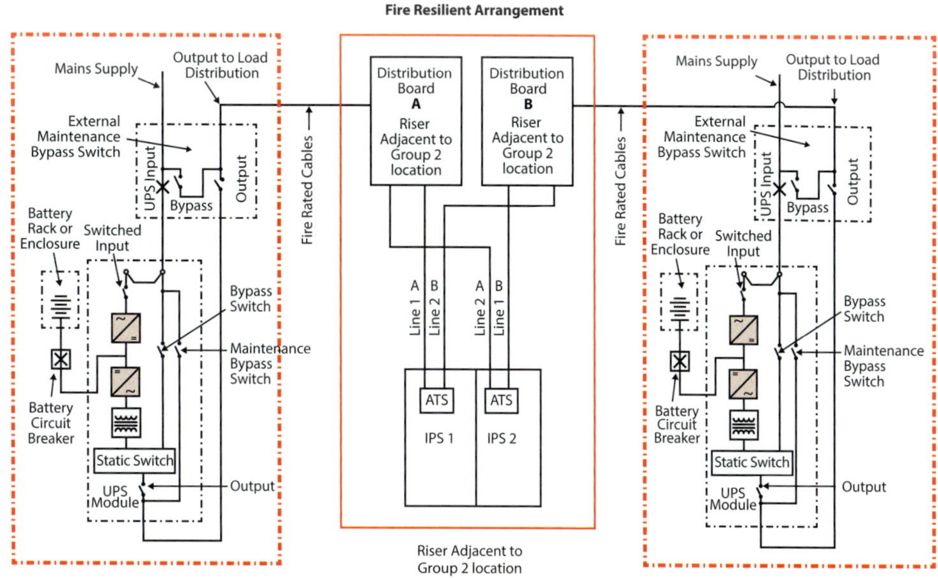

In Figure 9.3, it can be seen that, although there are two remote fire segregated UPS supplies from separate UPS configurations, where cabling leaves one protected area, passes through another compartment to get to a third compartment, it is possible for the effects of fire to affect the electrical supply to the medical IT system. This would create a loss of supply to the medical equipment and as such compromise the high dependency patient.

The potential loss of supply can be mitigated by the use of fire resistant distribution circuit cabling or other equivalent methods.

▼ **Figure 9.4** Medical IT system in separate fire compartment

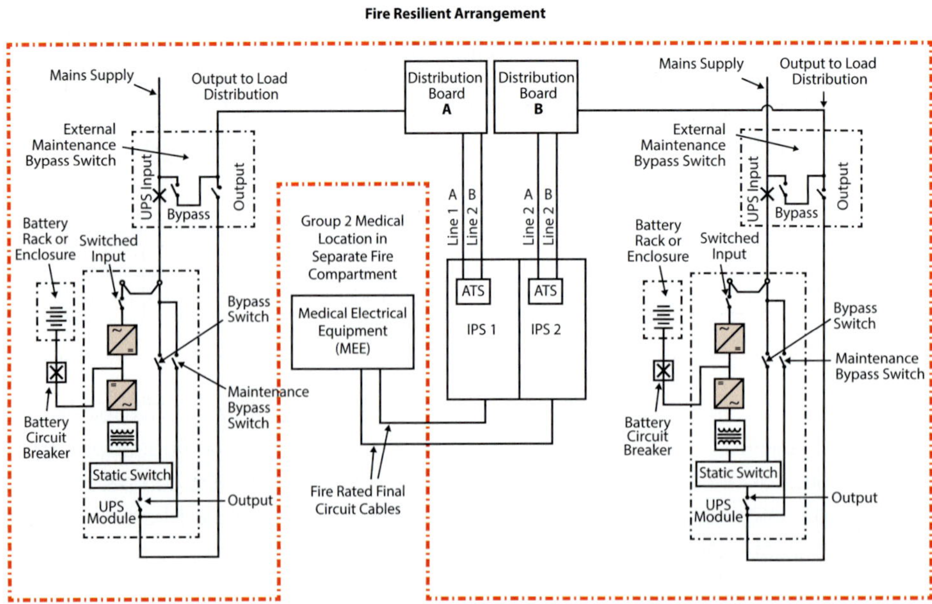

In Figure 9.4 the electrical supplies and medical IT system are located within one fire rated enclosure and the final circuits in a separate fire compartment. The cables pass through a third area that could be potentially be affected by fire, which would result in loss of individual final circuits and loss of power.

In order to mitigate the risk of loss of power, fire protected final circuit cabling should be applied.

Over-reliance on dated documents

It is important to note that by solely focusing on aged documentation and without considering the wider suite of documentation and having a general understanding of construction-related information, it is possible for the designer and installer to fail to meet the level of resilience and other site specific requirements.

Prior to revision, HTM 06-01 (2007) did not directly recognise the importance of fire rated cabling in circuits indicated above.

Groups 0, 1 and 2 medical locations are defined in international standards as well as in BS 7671. However, there is no direct comparison or alignment between the groups and the risk categories that are identified in both HTM and SHTM 06-01.

HTM 06-01 (2007) adds to the confusion by defining a Clinical Risk Category 4 area as an area for 'patients in special medical locations'. This mismatch can only be explained as a timing issue, as NHS Estates at the time (being an Executive Agency of the Department of Health), which later became incorporated into the Department of Health, was formulating the risk-based approach. This approach was not aligned with IEC 60364-7-710 and consequently the two systems were derived separately, and so provide two different perspectives.

Further examination of the HTM 06-01 approach reveals that clinical and business risk classifications appear to be more aligned with the types of electrical infrastructure, including HV systems that are outside the scope of BS 7671, that the healthcare premise operates and generally acknowledges the wider impact to the clinical and support services provided.

HTM 06-01A produces a risk matrix for designers, which is based on the use against the different formats of infrastructure that can be seen in UK healthcare premises.

▼ **Figure 10.1** Risk of electrical failure by infrastructure (from HTM 06-01, courtesy of the DoH)

RISK OF ELECTRICAL FAILURE BY INFRASTRUCTURE

Risk by clinical category (refer to Chapter 4 under 'Clinical risk')	Distribution strategy (refer to Chapter 6)				
	Primary supply: unified distribution (Fig.14)	Primary and secondary supply - unified and segregated distribution (Fig. 15)	Primary and secondary supply - unified and dual unified distribution (Fig. 16)	Dual-primary and dual-secondary supply - unified and dual-unified infrastructure (Fig. 17)	Dual primary and dual HV secondary supply - dual unified infrastructure (Fig. 18)
Life support complex surgery	HIGH	HIGH	SIGNIFICANT	MODERATE	LOW
Special medical locations	SIGNIFICANT	SIGNIFICANT	MODERATE	MODERATE	LOW
Emergency care and diagnostic	MODERATE	MODERATE	MODERATE	LOW	RESIDUAL
Ambulant care and diagnostic	MODERATE	MODERATE	LOW	LOW	RESIDUAL
Support services and circulation	LOW	LOW	RESIDUAL	RESIDUAL	RESIDUAL

The matrix identifies the residual risks as determined by the building use and reviews the type of electrical infrastructure required. As can be seen, even with highly resilient systems, certain procedures leave residual risk.

In order to further address this risk, other mitigation measures can be brought in to ensure the continuity of the supply. Examining the table shows that higher Risk Categories such as 4 and 5, with a dual unified primary and secondary supply with a dual unified distribution system leaves a small residual risk.

In order to further minimise this risk, additional systems and measures are required to improve reliability.

The electrical infrastructure generic flow diagram (see Figure 10.2) explains the use of systems for different clinical risk categories.

Although the risk categorization applied in HTM 06-01A does not figure in BS 7671, it has to be recognised that this type of risk analysis is a useful tool for determining the type of infrastructure that should be provided.

BS 7671 is often criticised for its lack of clear guidance, however, as a national wiring standard it cannot prescribe specific guidance. Documents such as HTMs and SHTMs are therefore invaluable in assisting the designer and installer (refer to Chapter 3 of HTM 06-01A).

▼ **Figure 10.2** Generic infrastructure flow diagram (from HTM 06-01, courtesy of the DoH)

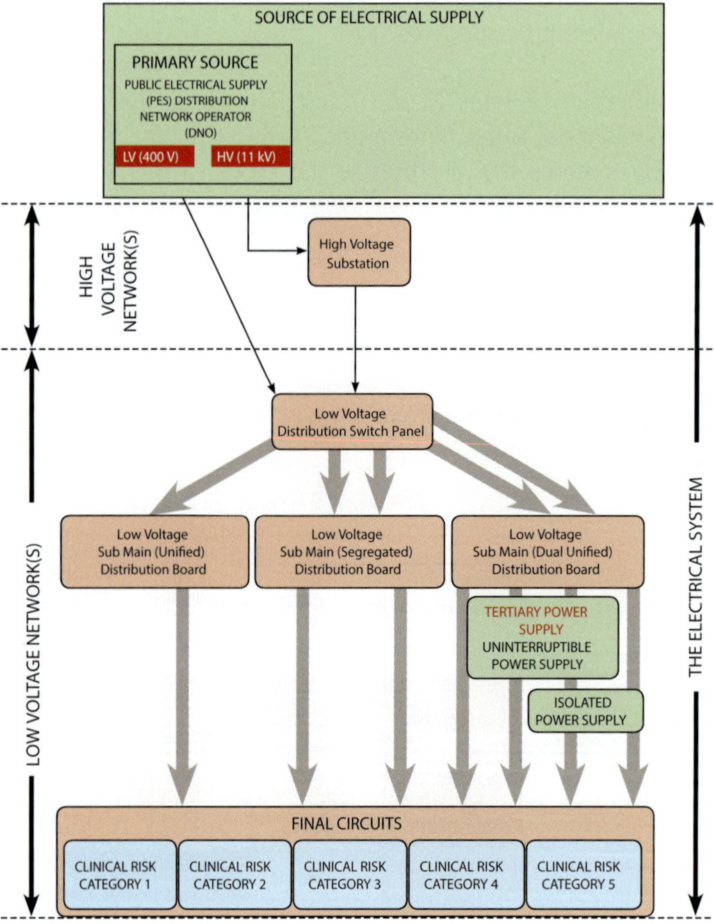

HTM 06-01 requires Risk Category 5 areas to have an N+1 arrangement, which is usually comprised of a second generator or, where the arrangement comprises of two duty sharing units to meet the load requirements, a third unit that will be available to minimise the impact or potential for failure (which may include failure to start) or added reliability during the maintenance of one unit.

Even with these measures in place, the risk matrix highlights that there is a residual risk with electrical infrastructure, regardless of the back-up infrastructure. However, by adding different layers of infrastructure, those critical areas with the most clinical risk can be targeted and the residual risk further reduced; this can be achieved by the addition of a tertiary power supply.

This requirement is indicated in the above electrical infrastructure generic flow diagram, which indicates that a Risk Category 4 area requires UPS to support some types of service that require a no-break supply. Due to the additional risk presented by a Risk Category 5 location, the diagram indicates that a medical IT system will be required.

10.1   Tertiary power supplies (TPS)

This type of power supply should not be considered as a long-term energy source in the same way that primary power or even secondary power units are. These supplies are usually only a means of bridging the gap between the failure of the primary power supply and the time required to bring the secondary supply (usually a generator) back online. Tertiary power supplies are generally used as a back-up supply for a given period of time, which is referred to as the 'autonomy time' of the system.

The autonomy time will depend on the type, capacity and number of cells in the battery string. The most commonly used are valve regulated lead acid (VRLA) batteries to the former standard of BS 6290-4 (1977). (Although still referenced by manufacturers in technical submissions, this standard has been replaced by BS EN 60896-21 and BS EN 60896-22). These types of batteries are more commonly known as sealed lead acid cells. The VRLA battery is a near-zero-gassing battery cell and hence presents a lower environmental hazard to the UPS room and surrounding area. With minimal gases emitted from the battery, there are usually no special ventilation requirements for the battery unit. However, ventilation and temperature control of some description will be required to keep the batteries within the optimum environmental conditions, enhance battery life and dispersal of any vapours/gases in accordance with the manufacturer's guidance.

In all instances it is the designer's responsibility to fully assess the need for ventilation and cooling for the particular installation. This assessment will need to take into account manufacturer recommendations and other factors including fire officer/fire safety adviser recommendations.

This type of battery comes with a ten-year design life, however, although the batteries will operate within a wide temperature differential, typically $-15\ °C$ to $+50\ °C$, they need to be maintained within a closer tolerance or their life expectancy and any warranty will be somewhat reduced.

10.2   Uninterruptable power supplies (UPS)

There are different types of UPS available on the market. A single conversion UPS is normally used in small personal computing or as a back-up for computerised processors. These units usually have an autonomy time of 30 minutes or less.

The double conversion UPS is more commonly used for medical systems. These systems are widely used as tertiary power supplies in healthcare applications.

▼ **Figure 10.3** Double conversion UPS arrangement

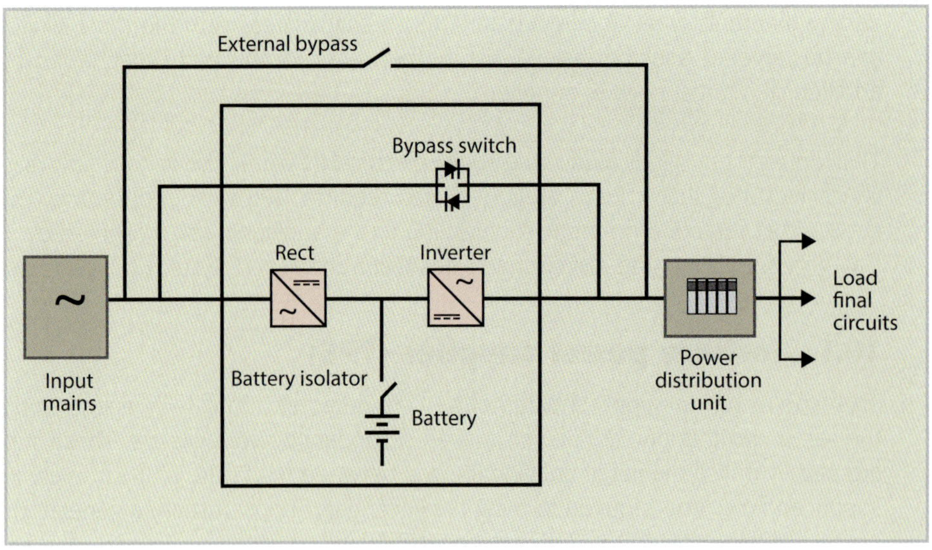

10.2.1 Other less widely used UPS in healthcare applications

Other less commonly used UPS include the hybrid topology double conversion on-demand UPS. These have a high efficiency as they work as an offline standby UPS. When power conditions fluctuate outside the pre-set conditions, the UPS switches to an online double conversion system.

The ferroresonant UPS operates in a similar way to the standby UPS with the exception that a ferroresonant transformer is used to filter the output. This transformer is designed to hold energy long enough to allow the UPS to switch the battery into circuit.

Rotary UPS is normally larger than other UPS and uses a high mass spinning flywheel to provide energy storage. The flywheel, due to the energy stored, is an excellent buffer against spike sags and other short-term power events. These types of UPS are mechanical units and will require regular maintenance to bearings etc.

10.2.2 Reliability of the UPS

The UPS may not necessarily be as reliable a piece of equipment as some might believe. Equipment manufacturers tend to indicate availability as:

$$\text{Availability} = \frac{\text{MTBF}}{\text{MTBF} + \text{MTTR}}$$

> **Note:**
> MTTF = Mean time to failure
> MTTR = Mean time to repair

Although this is represented in numbers of 9s, for example, 99.9992 % equating to 4.2 minutes of downtime per year, this has not allowed for maintenance, testing and recalibration which, without N+1 or similar arrangements, will bring down the availability figures.

In reality, the UPS may not have been maintained within the right parameters and, although the UPS electronics may meet those requirements, it is very likely that the UPS itself will not meet the reliability levels that may be expected by simply applying the availability formula.

Historically, transformer-based UPS were often more reliable forms of double conversion units. However, due to expense they were limited to larger units.

▼ **Figure 10.4** Transformer based UPS configuration

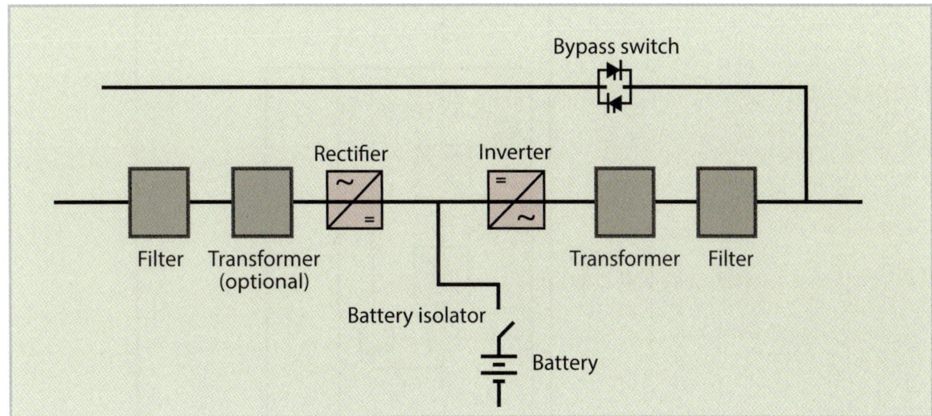

Transformerless units are now commonplace and their reliability has improved. They also have advantages in terms of weight and cost.

10.3 Safe approach to tertiary supplies

Although high availability factors are quoted, the reliability of the UPS supply should always be considered an ultimate last resort. As the battery can affect output, care should be taken by those owning and operating tertiary power supplies to ensure that the units are maintained correctly and the performance of the battery systems under duress are in line with expectations. For example, if clinicians believe they have a 1-hour battery back-up they must have that level of autonomy time; any degradation in battery autonomy time is not just an estate matter, it is a clinical matter as it affects the risk assessments that were put into place at the time of clinical commissioning.

10.4 Tertiary supply resilience

The following diagrams indicate how simple measures can improve the overall availability of the supplies.

Within medical locations, the primary requirement for uninterrupted power to life support and other vital ME equipment is to enable the generator to start and to pick up the supply from the point at which the mains failed.

Regulation 710.560.6.1.2 of BS 7671 allows the autonomy of the batteries in a UPS to be reduced from 3 hours to 1 hour, provided that the generator is able to take up the load within 15 s. This differs from the requirement in HTM 06-01 (2007), which allows some non-theatre areas to have a smaller autonomy time. It should be noted that the reduction stated in Regulation 710.560.6.1.2 does not apply to theatre lighting tertiary power supplies.

HTM 06-01 (2007) also indicates that the cascading UPS arrangement is as being a highly resilient arrangement. However, it should be noted that as the HTM is now dated there have been a number of technological advances. The developments in technology now mean that other combinations of these devices can be considered as having the same, if not more, resilience.

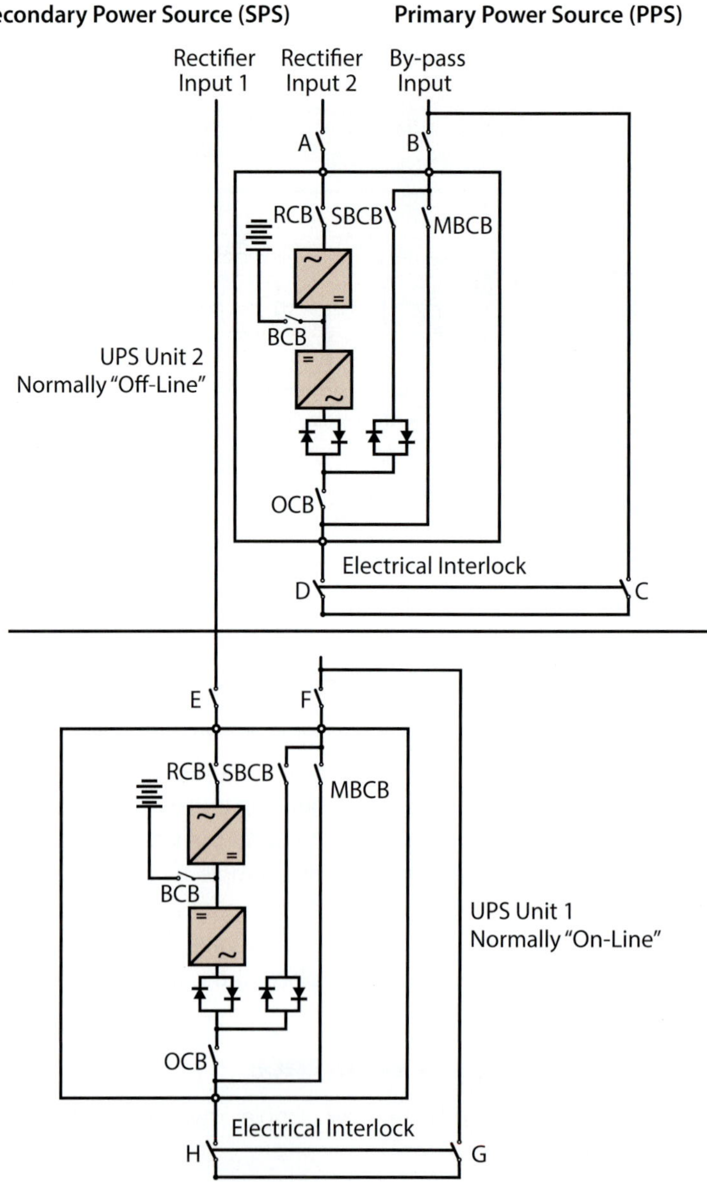

UPS-Basic Cascade Arrangement Indicated in HTM06-01A

This arrangement is now less common and is considered by the UPS industry as a 'legacy' arrangement with arrangements now consisting of two single UPS with automatic changeover or N+1 configurations.

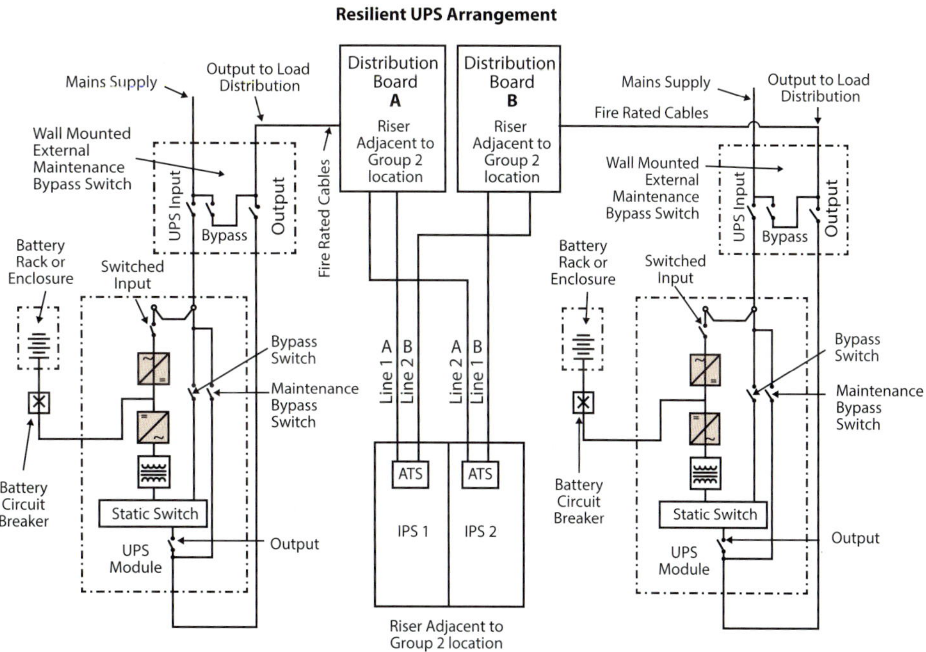

▼ Figure 10.6 Typical resilient UPS arrangement

UPS unit resilience can be enhanced by adding redundant parallel configurations.

This can be further enhanced by adding the external bypass. It should be noted that the bypass configuration indicated in this Guide may not be appropriate for all UPS modules, which may require additional interfaces or switching procedures to prevent damage or danger.

This can be further enhanced by adding the external bypass.

10.5 UPS fault levels and supply impedance

When selecting a UPS it is important to recognise that the fault level quoted by most UPS manufacturers is normally with the automatic internal bypass taking the load. This is acceptable in most instances except under mains failure conditions, which is the very reason for the use of a UPS. When specifying a UPS it is important to understand the fault levels and hence fault clearing capabilities when on battery only.

There are UPS available that are able to deliver both the correct line impedance to allow imaging to function and the protection to operate properly. However, where disconnection times cannot be achieved, applying the measures set out in Regulation 411.3.2.6 can often be used to achieve compliance.

In terms of imaging quality and supply impedance, this can sometimes involve the use of UPS inverters which have been specially 'tuned' to ensure that the correct values on battery only (off mains and bypass) are delivered. This usually involves oversizing of the inverter unit. Examples of this have been used on imaging systems involving 80 kVA UPS with components that are more often seen in 250 kVA units.

10.6 Improving the resilience of IT systems

Unlike HTM guidance, it is important to note that neither the international standard HD 60364-7-710:2012 or BS 7671 require the use of a UPS to support a medical IT system.

Changeover devices that allow different supplies to be switched in have been developed by manufacturers. These include the SATS by Starkstrom and the ATICS by Bender.

▼ **Figure 10.7** Examples of changeover devices (Images courtesy of Bender, Socomec and Starkstrom)

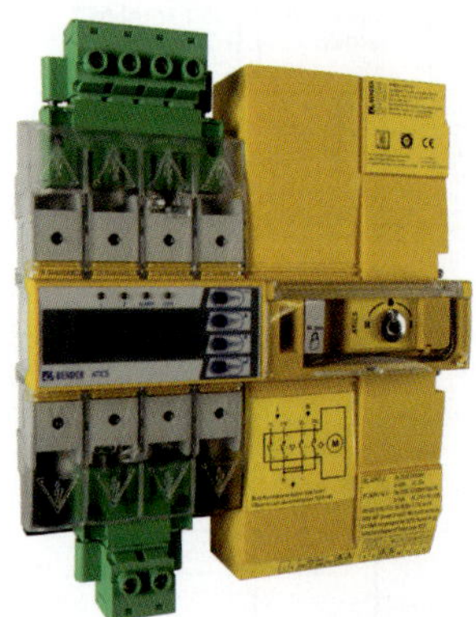

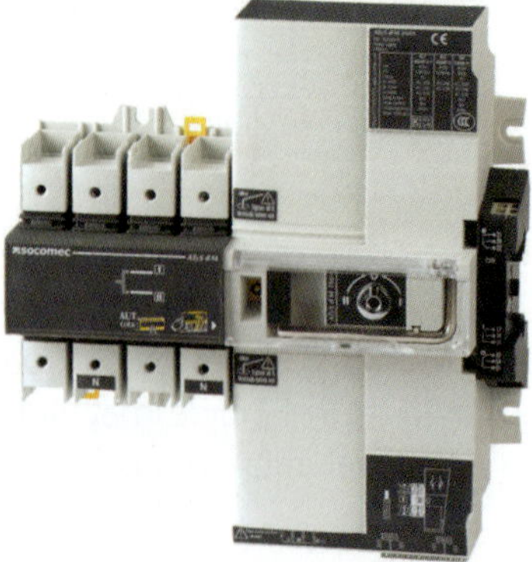

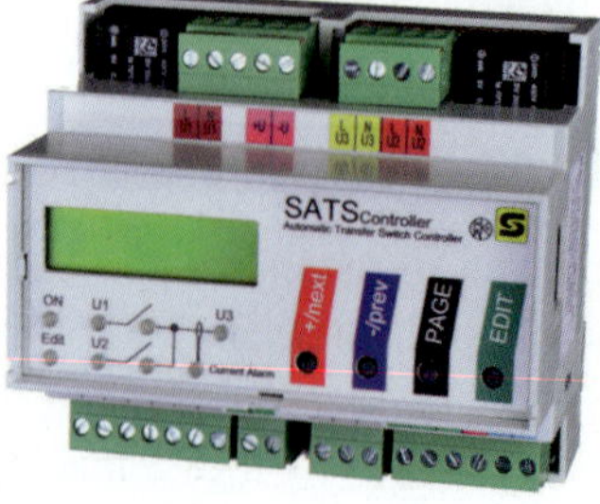

These units allow additional switching of the power supplies so that the availability of power is kept where it is needed.

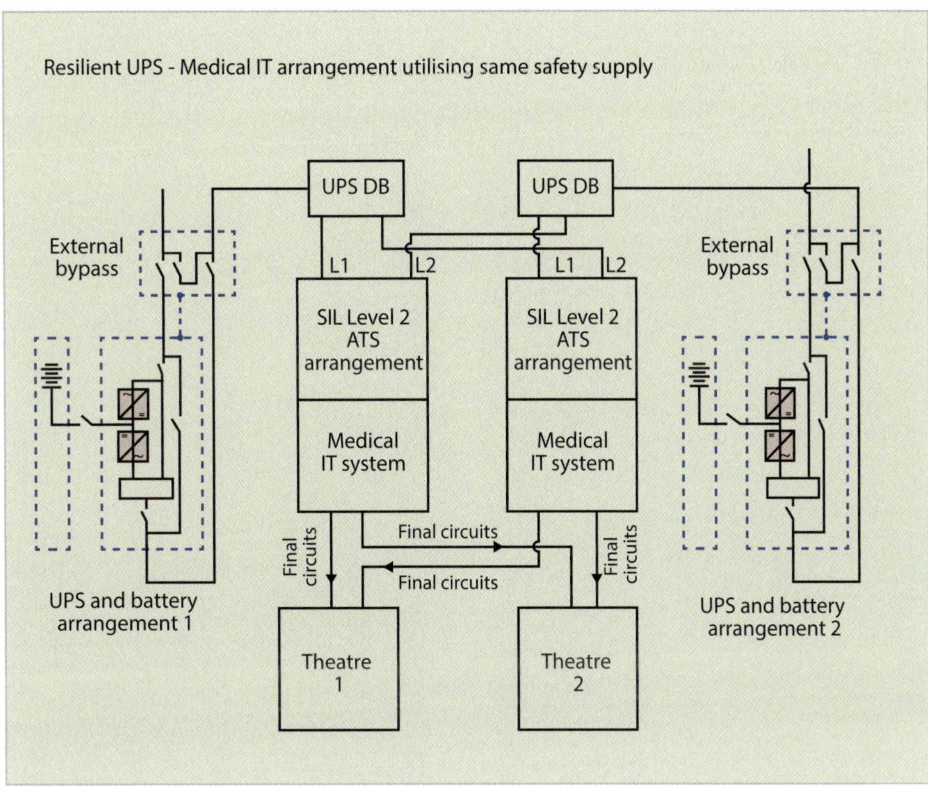

Enhancing the resilience of the changeover units can be provided by examining the reliability of the components in terms of mechanical, electrical and control systems reliability, and thereafter looking at the effects of faults and component replacement strategies. There is a system of measurement of this sort of criteria in many industries, including process, petrochemical and nuclear industries.

This system is based on the international standard IEC EN 61508. In the UK, this is recognised through a compliant process through the BS EN 61508 series of documents and is identified as a safety integration level (SIL) rating. It is important to note that there is currently no SIL standard requirement for healthcare and neither the HTM guidance nor BS 7671 requires this. However, the minimum requirement set out in BS 7671 is that changeover units comply with BS EN 60947-6-1.

The electrical engineer looking to design a medical location is not generally expected to know about SIL ratings, especially as it is not a Section 710 requirement. However, a SIL rating is an actual measure of the overall safety function being performed by a specific safety system. While there are SIL standards for nuclear and rail etc., there are no standards that are particular to healthcare.

SIL ratings are based on a series of levels 1-4, with 4 being the most dependable and 1 being the least.

SIL is defined as a relative level of risk reduction provided by a safety function, or to specify a target level of risk reduction, in a system or device. In simple terms, SIL is a measurement of performance required for a safety instrumented function (SIF).

SIL is a simple numbering system, based on BS EN 61508, that sets out the safety criteria for a device. It is based around the requirements for hardware safety integrity, which are based on a probabilistic analysis of the device.

Mathematical probability

Probability of failure on demand (PFD) and risk reduction factor (RRF) of low demand operation for different SILs as defined in IEC EN 61508 are as follows:

SIL	PFD	PFD (power)	RRF
1	0.1-0.01	$10^{-1} - 10^{-2}$	10-100
2	0.01-0.001	$10^{-2} - 10^{-3}$	100-1000
3	0.001-0.0001	$10^{-3} - 10^{-4}$	1000-10,000
4	0.0001-0.00001	$10^{-4} - 10^{-5}$	10,000-100,000

In continuous operation the relevant parameters are:

SIL	PFD	PFD (power)	RRF
1	0.00001-0.000001	$10^{-5} - 10^{-6}$	100,000-1,000,000
2	0.000001-0.0000001	$10^{-6} - 10^{-7}$	1,000,000-10,000,000
3	0.0000001-0.00000001	$10^{-7} - 10^{-8}$	10,000,000-100,000,000
4	0.00000001-0.000000001	$10^{-8} - 10^{-9}$	100,000,000-1,000,000,000

SIL ratings are not just mathematical calculations based on the probability of a product or systems failure. To achieve a SIL rating a rigorous process is needed and all parts of BS EN 61508 will need to be considered. This consists of the following:

Part 1:   General requirements

Part 2:   Requirements for electrical/electronic/programmable electronic safety-related systems

Part 3:   Software requirements

Part 4:   Definitions and abbreviations

Part 5:   Examples of methods for the determination of safety integrity levels

Part 6:   Guidelines on the application of Parts 2 and 3

Part 7:   Overview of techniques and measures

The flow chart below is an extract from BS EN 61508-1 2010 that sets out the overall safety cycle from concept to decommissioning.

▼ **Figure 11.1** Overall safety lifecycle

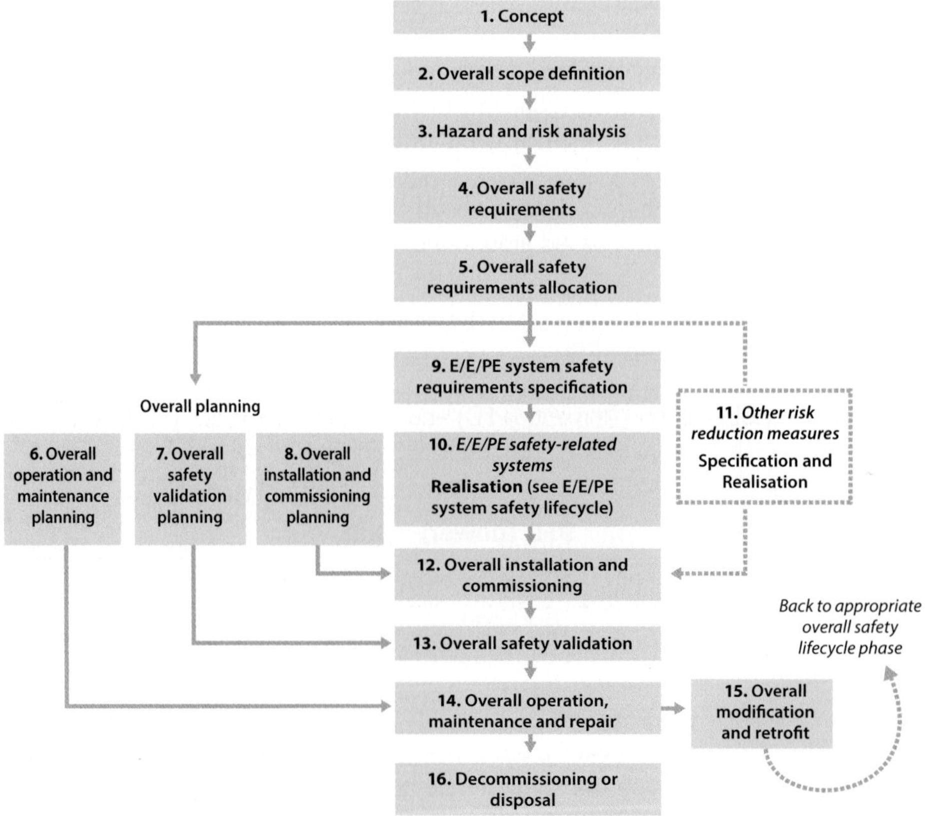

A SIL rating applies to an entire system, not just to a component within a system, as individual products or components do not have SIL ratings.

SIL ratings are used when implementing a SIF that must reduce an existing intolerable process risk level to a tolerable risk level.

11.1   SIL certification

BS EN 61508-1 2010 does not specify the requirement for a SIL certificate; it does, however, require a functional safety assessment to be carried out.

Functional safety is only achieved by designing, planning, developing, commissioning, operating and making changes (as necessary during the design and testing process) during the lifetime of the system, including decommissioning/replacing after a product has reached its end of life.

Many certificates relate to individual devices, SIL ratings are meant to look at the system, from sensor to actuator. Consequently, to have a SIL rating for a particular device slightly masks the resulting statement, as it is purely dependent on the conditions under which it has been made.

In order to be compliant with the standards, it is up to the user to ensure that procedures have been followed properly, that the proof testing is conducted correctly, and that suitable documentation of the design, process, and procedures exists.

The process by which the functional safety assessment has been conducted should comply with the BS EN 61508 series of documents in terms of the independence, competence and the procedures of the assessment body.

It is worth noting that any certification body that has the relevant parts of BS EN 61508 within its scope of accreditation will ensure that correct certification is in place.

11.1.1   Selecting equipment

The equipment or system must be used in the manner in which it was intended in order to successfully obtain the desired risk reduction level. Just buying SIL 2 or SIL 3 suitable components does not ensure a SIL 2 or SIL 3 system.

11.2   Enhancement of standard automatic transfer

An enhancement to the standard transfer switch is necessary in order to meet the requirements of SIL.

Functional safety does not mean that a device developed in accordance with the rules of functional safety can be operated longer than a device where such measures were not applied. Meaning that a device or system can be operated with a high grade of functional safety during its described useful lifetime.

Currently, the ATICS by Bender has achieved the SIL 2 standard for reliability and safety in line with IEC EN 61508 although at the time of publication other devices are believed to be undergoing SIL accreditation processes.

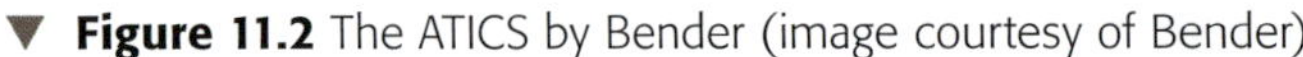

▼ **Figure 11.2** The ATICS by Bender (image courtesy of Bender)

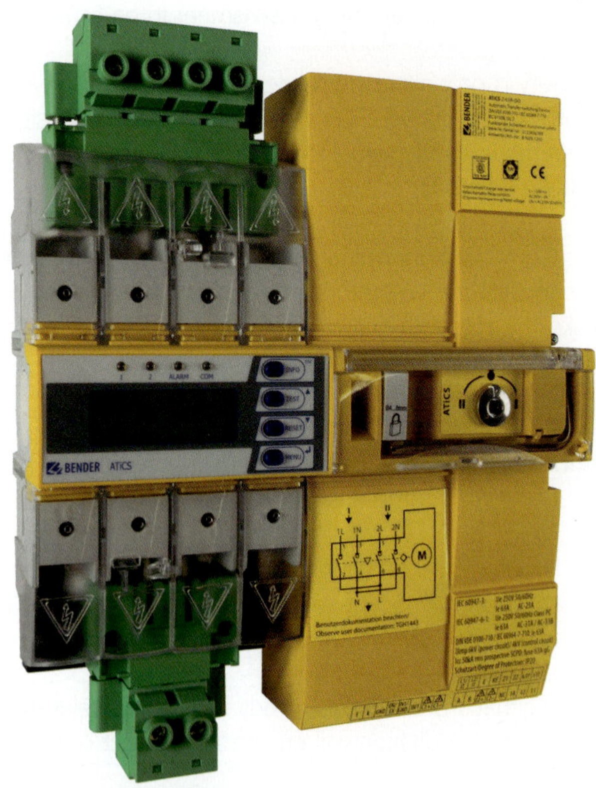

As part of the overall planning and design processes to achieve SIL, designers and developers are required to include the safe operation of the system by the user, for example, correct reaction in case of an alarm, which will need to include adequate training of the end user and also ensuring that maintenance regimes are in place.

It is important to remember that, despite all the checks and systems in place, nobody can prevent a component from failing. Failures can be detected by integral monitoring causing an alarm to be generated where a fault has been detected, thereby, allowing the user to obtain information about the failure so that action can be taken rather than just observing a malfunction.

Theatre operating lights {#12}

The importance of theatre operating lighting cannot be over-stressed.

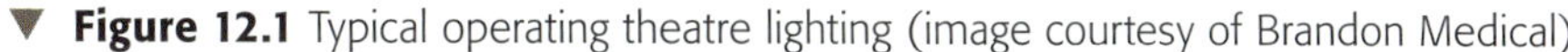

▼ **Figure 12.1** Typical operating theatre lighting (image courtesy of Brandon Medical)

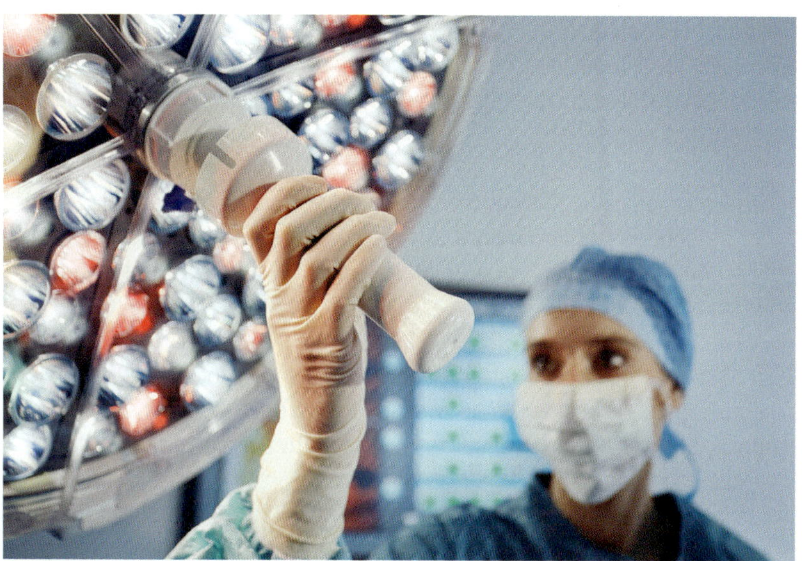

The theatre lighting system is sometimes misunderstood with some designers believing that the battery autonomy time in the medical IT system is linked.

HTM 06-01A, BS 7671 Regulation 710.560.6.1.1 (i) and BS EN 60601-2-41 require an autonomy time of at least 3 hours. Although BS 7671 does not detail further requirements, it is both an HTM requirement and standard practice that each theatre has its own rectifier unit.

Theatre lighting is actually an ELV system and is restricted to 25 V AC or 60 V DC, so there has to be consideration with respect to the location of the batteries and rectifier with the actual length of run of the cables.

The 2007 version of HTM 06-01 refers to these supplies as being SELV. However, the same documentation requires the metalwork of the operating light to be bonded to the electrical system. As SELV systems have no direct connection to earth, a system with such a connection would be outside the requirements of SELV and would be more aligned to that of a PELV system. As with all equipment, manufacturer instructions and requirements should be consulted before installation and connection to the fixed electrical installation.

▼ **Figure 12.2** PELV configuration

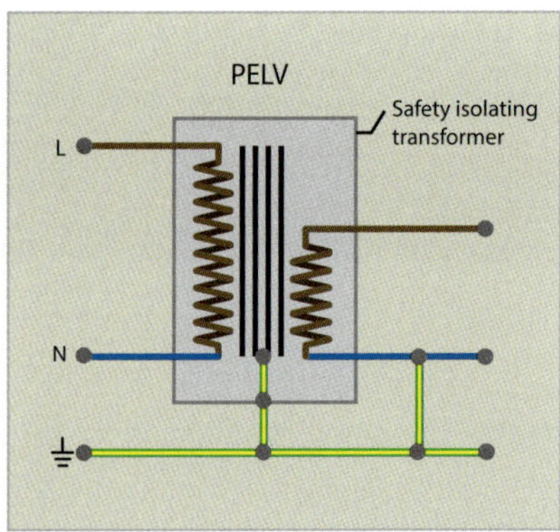

Historically, halogen lighting could be in the order of 600 W, however, with the influx of modern LED lighting the size of the load has fallen away dramatically. This means that battery loads and sizes have been reduced to a more manageable size. The units are normally located in rooms adjacent to the theatre, for example, in dirty corridors and utility rooms, etc.

As these units get moved away from the load for spatial or aesthetic reasons, designers should be cautious of the impact to the resilience and functionality of the light when locating the PELV tertiary power supply unit away from the medical location by architects etc.

Whilst distance from the battery unit in terms of functionality may only a matter of increasing the cross sectional area of the cables to allow for volt drop and fault clearance, there is a fundamental resilience matter to consider.

One of the fundamental principles of resilience, which is described earlier in Section 8, is the removal of the single point of failure. Moving the tertiary supply batteries and inverter unit away from the point of use increases the likelihood of that failure.

Generally, the inverter unit to the theatre light will be 'dual fed' with a supply and an alternative supply to the battery unit. However, in the unlikely event of a total power failure to the supply and its back-up, for example, the generators failing to start or a major fault in the network, the tertiary power supply system will power the PELV theatre light for a minimum period of three hours.

Where the battery unit is 'remote' from the source, for example, in a plant-room above the theatre or along a corridor and away from the room it is supplying, there is an inherent risk of failure from an external influence such as fire or mechanical damage. In the case of fire occurring in the room where the batteries are located or where the cables pass through en route to the theatre light, there is no other form of back-up or redundancy of lights, etc., the theatre light is lost and the theatre staff are left to complete the procedures by hand-held or head-mounted torches or to relocate to another theatre (if one is available), which is less than satisfactory for all concerned.

In order to mitigate this potential failure, a reasonable step may be to protect the enclosure in which the battery unit is located from fire (i.e. fire separated from the plant in the plantroom). Additionally, any supply cables from the battery and rectifier unit and the light source should be with PH120 fire-rated cable, which should preferably be armoured or protected from mechanical damage.

PH120 cabling only provides a level of protection for two hours, and any enclosure for the battery unit would require an appropriate level of fire protection depending on position and construction. Although the battery autonomy time is three hours, this does, however, provide a similar level of service in a fire condition. This is because the hazard of losing light due to loss of power is different to that of the effects of fire. Despite additional fire and smoke protection in this type of area, it would be unlikely that any area would have three hours fire separation. Consequently, as part of the fire safety procedures and protocols, action would have to be taken, i.e. to evacuate or move to another theatre block if the operation had to continue before the structural fire precautions fail.

Given the importance of a operating light it is reasonable to ensure two-hour fire protection and fire separation of the unit from the other plant. Whilst this Guide does not advocate variation from the planning requirements set out in the HTMs and Health Building Note (HBNs) published by the Department of Health, it does look to be cognisant of the impact so as to innovate and counteract the impact of derogations where they have been applied.

Generator supplies 13

Generators form an important part of hospital electrical supplies and are used for emergency standby both at LV and HV levels depending on the hospital infrastructure design philosophy. They can also be used as a form of peak or load lopping by operating the unit(s); this is usually during synchronised mode with the mains.

Alternative forms of load lopping are usually found in low or zero carbon technologies, such as photovoltaic (PV) or combined heat and power (CHP). However, CHP should not be considered an emergency standby or safety power supply as the set-up of these units is for energy reduction and not primarily for safety services.

Historically, CHP units were usually sized on the heat output requirements so that the heating/hot water loads are satisfied, however, the CHP can be configured to have an electrical lead function which is commonplace today.

The difficulty with CHP units is that they are designed to be operated in line with Engineering Requirements G59, which usually means that, if there is a disturbance on the system, the CHP electrical supply is switched out through the 'G59 relay'.

The standard by which generators were historically specified was Model Engineering Specification (MES) C44 (published by the Department of Health). This set out the minimum parameters and requirements for generator specification. This standard was last updated in 1997 and is now out of step with generator technology and the needs of modern health care installations.

In terms of secondary sources of supply, generator supplies are considered to be reliable, available to accept 60 % of the load within 15 s and take up the rest of the load in 20 s, which was an MES C44 requirement.

BS 7671:2008+A3(2015) Regulation 551.4 requires that "fault protection shall be provided for the installation in respect of each source of supply or combination of sources of supply that can operate independently of other sources or combination of sources …".

In effect, this means that each method of supply shall be capable of operating and, if necessary, disconnecting the supply in each relevant arrangement, i.e. on mains supply, generator supply as an alternative and, finally, in synchronised mode where applicable.

Most designers are familiar with designing electrical protection using the electrical distribution system. However, what is not fully appreciated is the difference between two electricity sources that are the same size. Often, generator protection is set using relatively low earth fault settings to ensure protection is achieved for the cables when on generator supplies.

In many instances, an alternative or emergency supply is required to keep operations going despite an adverse incident, such as the loss of electricity supply. A safety supply with a very sensitive setting may well be acceptable from a cable or fault level protection point of view, but is of little use when, the moment you require your emergency supply, it trips on a small level of earth fault current due to sensitive protection settings.

It is therefore important to look at the secondary power supply protection settings to ensure that the protection operates in accordance with the secondary supply intent.

This surety of supply requirement will mean an assessment of the generator characteristics, which will in turn require an assessment of the load characteristics against the generator parameters. This assessment will need to consider engine and alternator rating, step load acceptance in conjunction with the type of load that is to be applied. When sizing a generator, standard steady state loads can be relatively simplistic, it is common that a load profile may consist of many types of complex loads.

For example, if the load profile should consist of one (or several) motor components then inrush currents of generally 6 times nominal load values can be expected. These need to be considered along with any locked rotor requirements. The upshot of all this can result in a much larger generator than is actually needed to accommodate the much lower normal running currents required once the inrush phase has passed. This in turn can be problematic as generators should be run above 33 % loading to ensure that they are engaged enough to avoid coking of cylinders. To avoid the 'inrush issue' soft start mechanisms could be employed where possible.

Additionally, an assessment of the amount of variable speed controllers, UPS equipment as a percentage of the full load current should be made. These considerations, once fully assessed, are then normally followed by fuel type choice, sound levels and cost issues.

13.1 Generator ratings

Generating sets meeting the requirements of the Standard ISO 8528-1 are used to generate electrical power for continuous, peak-load and standby applications. The classifications within the Standard are as follows:

Standby power rating

In ISO 8528-1, this is referred to as emergency standby power (ESP) and is defined as: "...the maximum power available during a variable electrical power sequence, under the stated operating conditions, for which a generating set is capable of delivering in the event of a utility power outage or under test conditions for up to 200 h of operation per year with the maintenance intervals and procedures being carried out as prescribed by the manufacturers."

Prime power rating

Prime power is defined in ISO 8528-1 as: "...the maximum power which a generating set is capable of delivering continuously whilst supplying a variable electrical load when operated for an unlimited number of hours per year under the agreed operating conditions with the maintenance intervals and procedures being carried out as prescribed by the manufacturer."

There are separate requirements for indefinite and limited time power requirements.

Constant power rating

Continuous power is defined in ISO 8528-1 as: "...the maximum power which the generating set is capable of delivering continuously whilst supplying a constant electrical load when operated for an unlimited number of hours per year under the agreed operating conditions with the maintenance intervals and procedures being carried out as prescribed by the manufacturer."

From a design and specification point of view, the designer should be aware of the limitations of specifying standby or prime power ratings. Additionally, the designer should be aware of the effective uplift in generator size so as to comply with constant power rating. Generators for safety services are required by Regulation 560.6.13 of BS 7671 and require generating sets used as a safety source to comply with BS 7698-12.

Looking at wider compatibility issues of the system, such as the circuit-breakers and cable selection for the emergency generators, is normally secondary or often not given the consideration that it is due. As these 'emergencies' may include fire situations, it is important to ensure that the generator and alternative supplies are segregated from the normal supply.

If the service includes fire protection activities, such as a fire fighter or evacuation lift, the electrical supplies will need to be designed, selected, installed and commissioned in accordance with BS 8519.

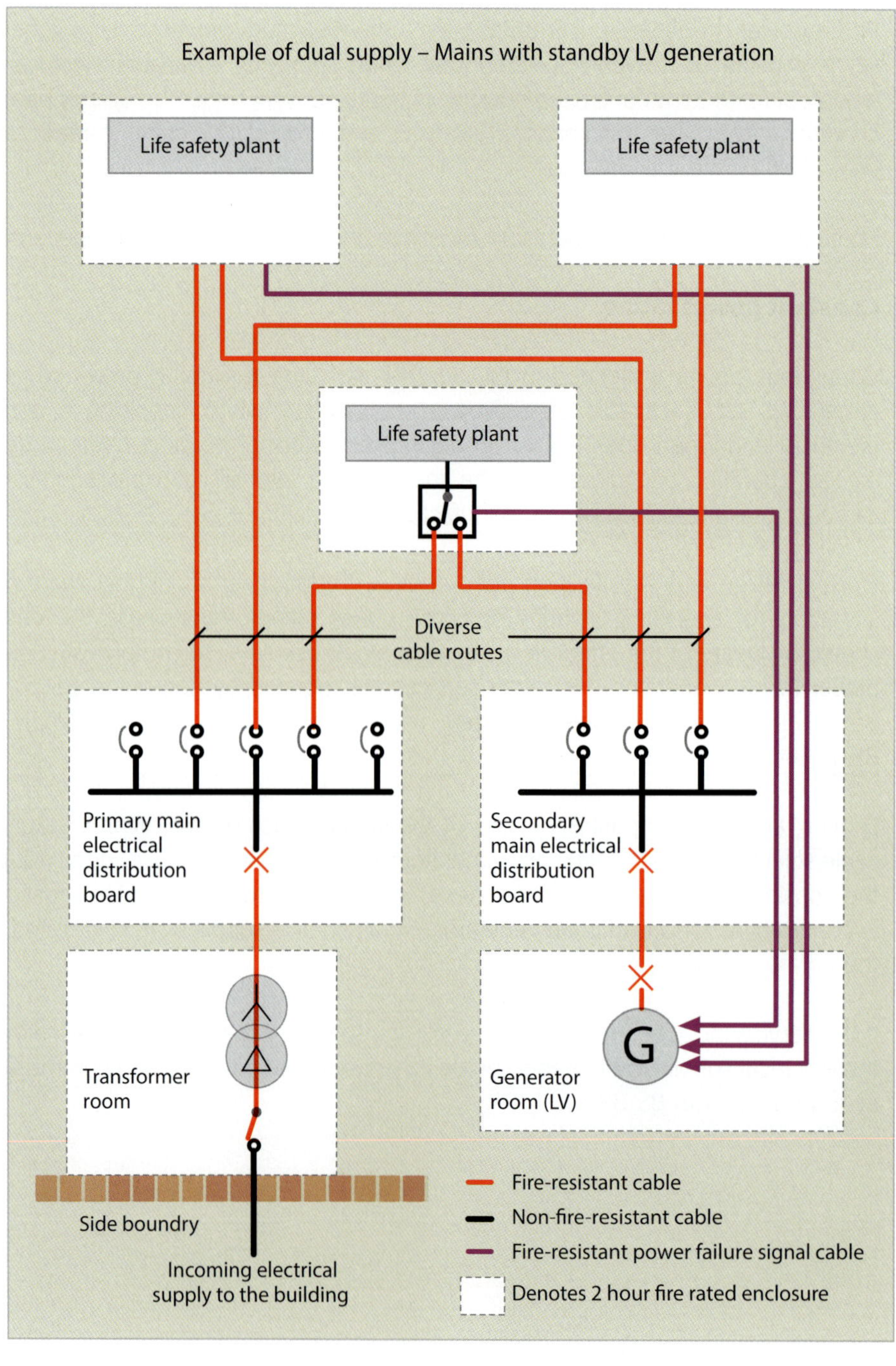

▼ **Figure 13.1** Example of dual supply – mains standby LV generation

The use of the generator as an emergency supply is very different from the electrical supply of the same size which is obtained from the DNO. The DNO supply is assumed to have an incredibly large power source at primary level, whereas the diesel generator is effectively a large engine similar to a truck engine with an alternator attached, where the speed can be temporarily affected by load. Consequently, common sense would dictate that the mains supply can deliver a larger fault level than such an engine and alternator arrangement. However, when choosing circuit-breakers, the designer must be aware that a generator is able to deliver extremely large fault levels for a very short period of time; in some cases this value can be up to 10 times the nominal current rating but will quickly degrade.

Further details relating to fault levels in generators can be found in Appendix 3.

Generally, in medical locations, the principal method of protection against electric shock is automatic disconnection of supply (ADS). Part of meeting the requirements for fault protection is the requirement for protective bonding. This approach requires exposed and extraneous-conductive-parts to be connected with the main earthing terminal (MET).

The general requirements of BS 7671 apply to most installations including Group 0 medical locations. An extract of Table 41.1 is provided below indicating automatic disconnection in case of a fault for different voltages.

▼ **Table 14.1**   Extracted from Table 41.1 (BS 7671)

System	$50\,V < U_0 \leq 120\,V$ (seconds)		$120\,V < U_0 \leq 230\,V$ (seconds)		$230\,V < U_0 \leq 400\,V$ (seconds)		$U_0 > 400\,V$ (seconds)	
	AC	DC	AC	DC	AC	DC	AC	DC
TN	0.8	NOTE	0.4	5	0.2	0.4	0.1	0.1
TT	0.3	NOTE	0.2	0.4	0.07	0.2	0.04	0.1

> **Note:** Disconnection is not required for protection against electric shock but may be required for other reasons, such as protection against thermal effects.

In Groups 1 and 2 medical locations, the maximum disconnection times are amended as follows:

▼ **Table 14.2**   Extracted from Table 710 (BS 7671)

System	$25\,V < U_0 \leq 50\,V$ (seconds)		$50\,V < U_0 \leq 120\,V$ (seconds)		$120\,V < U_0 \leq 230\,V$ (seconds)		$230\,V < U_0 \leq 400\,V$ (seconds)		$U_0 > 400\,V$ (seconds)	
	AC	DC	AC	DC	AC	DC	AC	DC	AC	DC
TN	5	5	0.3	2	0.3	0.5	0.05	0.06	0.02	0.02
TT	5	5	0.15	0.2	0.05	0.1	0.02	0.06	0.02	0.02

> **Note:** In TN systems, a value of 25 V AC or 60 V DC may be met with protective equipotential bonding if it complies with the disconnection time in accordance with Table 710.

Table 14.2 is a modified version of Table 710 in BS 7671, which gives maximum disconnection times for system and voltages. The note below the table reminds the reader that the 25 V AC or 60 V DC values are the important components for the disconnection time specified, which is dependent on the neutral earthing arrangement and voltage to earth (U_0).

This table is often misread. The particular area that applies to most installations is the column headed '**120 V < U_0 < 230 V**', as this heading refers to U_0, the nominal voltage to earth. However, it is often misread by those looking at 3-phase systems even though a standard 3-phase system U_0 is only 230 V, resulting in a misunderstanding of the actual disconnection time required.

▼ **Table 14.3** TT and TN disconnection times

System	120 V < U_0 ≤ 230 V	
	AC	DC
TN	0.3 s	0.5 s
TT	0.05 s	0.1 s

The above table applies to installations in Groups 1 and 2 medical locations, but does not apply to Group 0 medical locations – for such locations, the values of Table 41.1 would apply.

It should be noted that this is a variation from international standards where Table 41.1 applies for disconnection time for all medical locations. In other words, the UK has a slightly more onerous approach to disconnection times in medical locations than many of our European counterparts.

14.1 Simultaneously accessible exposed-conductive-parts

Regulation 710.411.3.2.5 also states that for TN, TT and IT systems, the voltage presented between simultaneously accessible exposed-conductive-parts and/or extraneous-conductive-parts shall not exceed 25 V AC or 60 V DC.

▼ **Figure 14.1** Simultaneously accessible exposed-conductive-parts

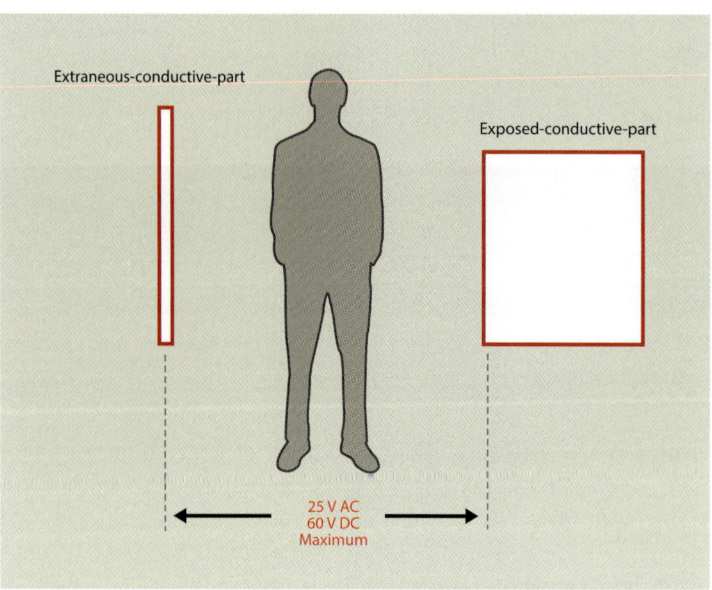

The permitted voltages presented between accessible parts for medical locations are reduced from 50 V AC or 120 V DC to 25 V AC or 60 V DC, This reduced value also affects the value of extra low voltage (ELV) applications, which are also 25 V AC or 60 V DC.

▼ **Figure 14.2** Application of equipotential bonding to reduce touch voltage

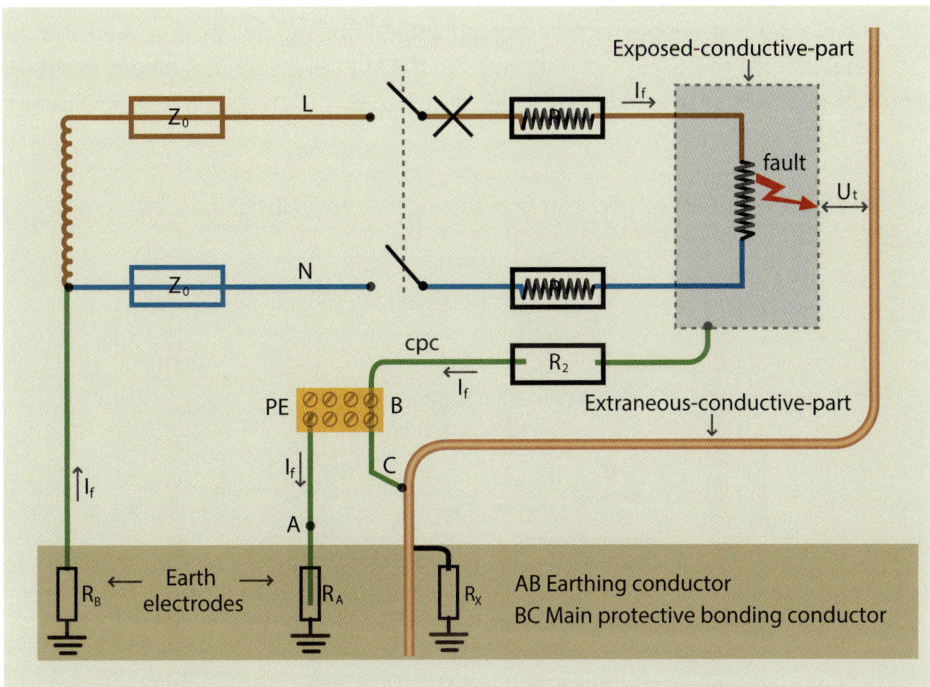

The application of touch voltage under earth fault conditions is indicated in this typical arrangement. This concept applies throughout Groups 1 and 2 medical locations, and should not be confused with any other concepts with voltages such as 10 mV, 50 mV or 100 mV – these are mentioned in MEIGaN (now withdrawn) and similar guidance.

14.2 Additional protection: supplementary equipotential

The concept of supplementary equipotential bonding can be found in the general requirements of BS 7671 and throughout the special locations sections (such as 702, 705 and 740) where additional protection is used extensively. The general principle is demonstrated below.

▼ **Figure 14.3** General principles of supplementary equipotential bonding

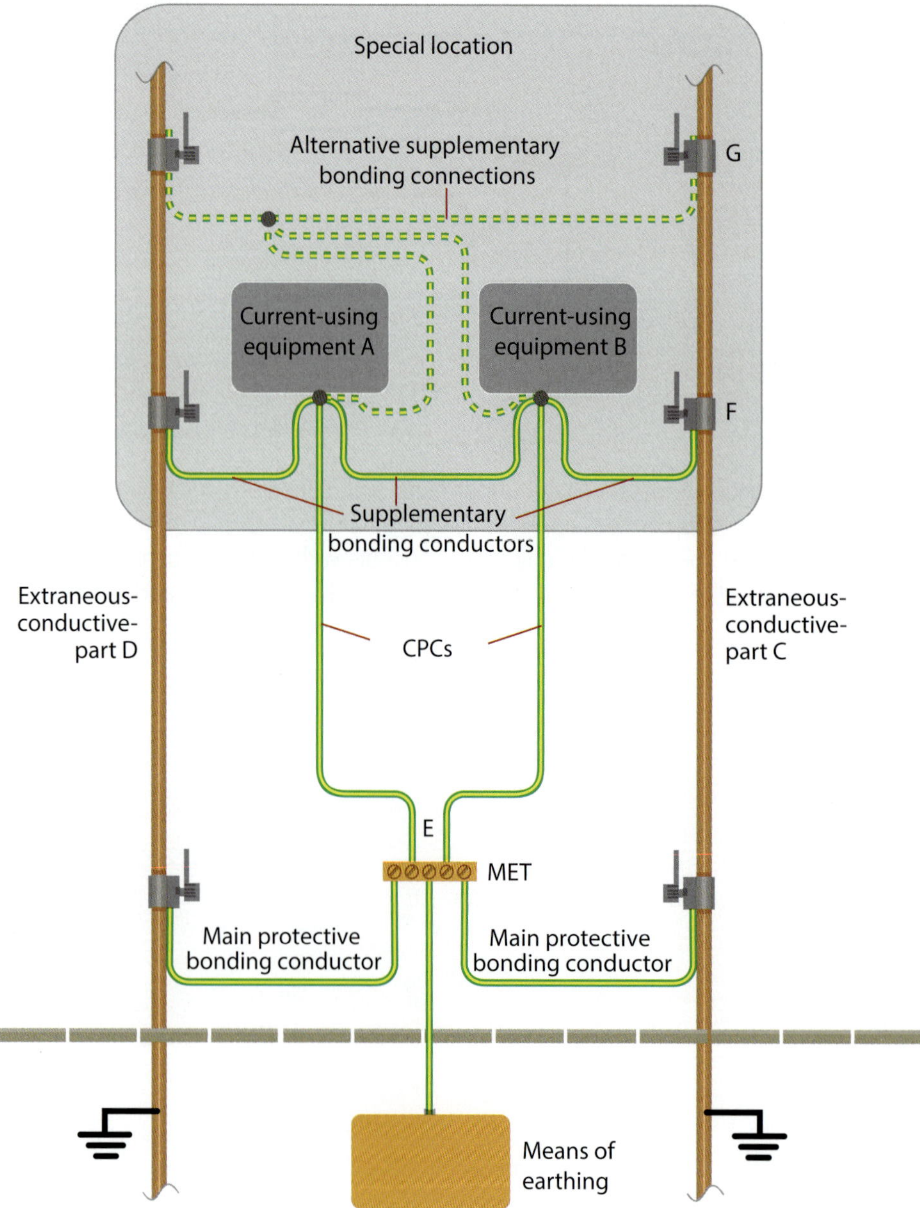

In medical locations there is a further augmentation of the requirements by requiring an equipotential bonding busbar (referred to in the UK as an EBB).

Regulation 710.415.2.1 requires that:

> *In each medical location of Group 1 and Group 2, supplementary equipotential bonding shall be installed and the supplementary equipotential bonding conductors shall be connected to the equipotential bonding busbar for the purpose of equalizing potential differences between the following parts, which are located or that may be moved into the "patient environment":*
>
> **(i)** *Protective conductors*
> **(ii)** *Extraneous-conductive-parts*
> **(iii)** *Screening against electrical interference fields, if installed*
> **(iv)** *Connection to conductive floor grids, if installed*
> **(v)** *Metal screens of isolating transformers, via the shortest route to the earthing conductor.*
>
> *Supplementary equipotential bonding connection points for the connection of ME equipment shall be provided in each medical location, as follows:*
> **(vi)** *Group 1: a minimum of one per patient location*
> **(vii)** *Group 2: a minimum of four but not less than 25 % of the number of medical IT socket-outlets provided per patient location.*
>
> > **Note:** *Fixed conductive non-electrical patient supports, such as operating theatre tables, physiotherapy couches and dental chairs should be connected to the equipotential bonding conductor unless they are intended to be isolated from earth.*

In order to satisfy the above requirements, it is necessary to design a supplementary equipotential bonding arrangement for each medical location.

There are various arrangements suggested by different sources not least those from MEIGaN that, despite its withdrawal, has left the industry with a legacy misunderstanding about supplementary equipotential bonding.

Examining the fundamental requirements of Regulation 710.415.2.1, it is necessary to provide supplementary equipotential bonding and additional supplementary equipotential bonding connection points. The number of connection points varies with respect to the different medical locations groups as per items (vi) and (vii) described above.

Figure 14.4 portrays the typical supplementary equipotential bonding requirements in a Group 1 medical location.

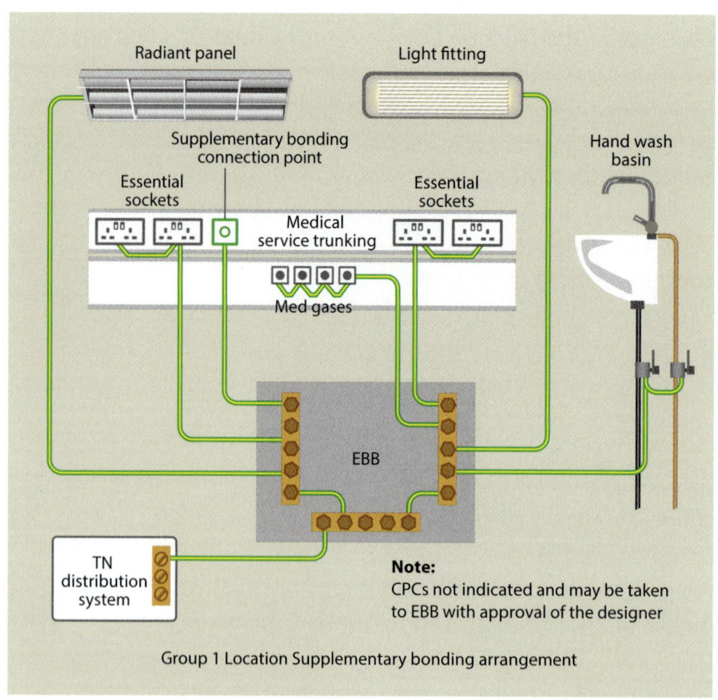

▼ Figure 14.4 Supplementary equipotential bonding to a Group 1 location

The size of conductors is limited by three factors:

(a) Regulation 544.2.3, which requires a minimum conductor size 2.5 mm² or 4 mm², if the conductor is unprotected;

(b) the resistance of the exposed-conductive-part to extraneous-conductive-part, as suggested in Regulation 710.415.2.2, which is not greater than 0.7 Ω in a Group 1 medical location; and

(c) the resulting voltage between simultaneously accessible parts, which, in accordance with Regulation 710.411.3.2.5, is 25 V AC or 60 V DC.

Even though we have been given a maximum value of 0.7 Ω in Regulation 710.415.2.2 this is not a performance criterion. There is still a requirement to satisfy touch voltage requirements of Regulation 710.411.3.2.5, which limits the touch voltage (U_L) on simultaneously accessible parts to 25 V AC or 60 V DC, which is a performance criterion.

In order to check this criterion has been met, the following formula will need to be applied.

For AC systems:

$$R_A \times I_a \leq 25 \text{ V}$$

Where:

R_A is the sum of the resistance in Ω of the earth electrode and protective conductor for the exposed-conductive-parts.

I_a is the fault current in A of the first fault of negligible impedance between a line conductor and an exposed-conductive-part. The value of I_a takes account of leakage currents and the total earthing impedance of the electrical installation.

Regulation 710.411.4 requires all TN final circuits up to 63 A in a Group 1 location to be protected by RCDs with an $I_{\Delta n}$ of 30 mA thereby limiting the value of current I_a.

Applying these values into the formula:

Touch voltage $= 0.7 \times 0.03 = 0.21$ V

The requirements for supplementary equipotential bonding are satisfied only when it has been established that the touch voltage is acceptable between simultaneously accessible exposed-conductive-parts and/or extraneous-conductive-parts, and the values given within Regulation 710.415.2.2 are not exceeded. In addition to the ohmic values, designers should be cognisant of the impact of long lengths of single cables passing through medical locations which may have an impact on EMC compliance.

In medical locations, rather than using an earthing terminal at the local distribution board to collect the protective conductors and supplementary equipotential bonding conductors, an equipotential bonding busbar (EBB) in the proximity of the location is used. This is effectively a local earth referencing/collection point within the medical location, providing supplementary equipotential bonding to exposed and extraneous conductors that should be fitted with (subject to shape and size) a BS 951 connector and label.

▼ **Figure 14.5** Warning label on BS 951 clamp

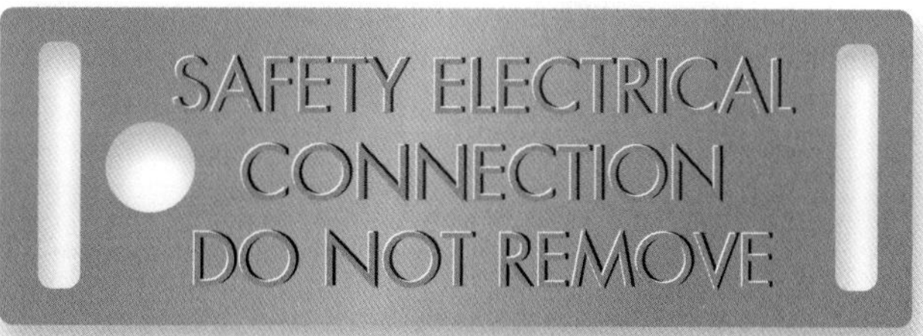

There are different arrangements which would meet the requirements of Section 710, in the Group 1 example above, the arrangement is strictly a supplementary equipotential bonding connection arrangement, whereby the relevant protective conductors from each circuit are simply bonded together at the EBB with a separate protective bonding conductor connected to the local distribution board.

Designers and installers are often challenged as to the location of EBBs, with architects unhappy at the sight of, or unable to aesthetically locate, these units. However, it is a regulatory requirement that the EBB is accessible.

Regulation 710.415.2.3 requires that "the equipotential bonding busbar shall be located in or near the medical location. Connections shall be so arranged that they are accessible, labelled, clearly visible and can easily be disconnected individually."

In order to meet this requirement, it is possible for contractors to construct their own EBB, although manufacturers have made their own version of the EBB for industry use. It should, however, be noted that non-proprietary units are less likely to be aesthetically acceptable to the architects or clients.

What is important to note is that the further away the EBB is situated from its point of use, the less effective it will be for its location type and may serve to increase EMC issues, such as noise or other signals.

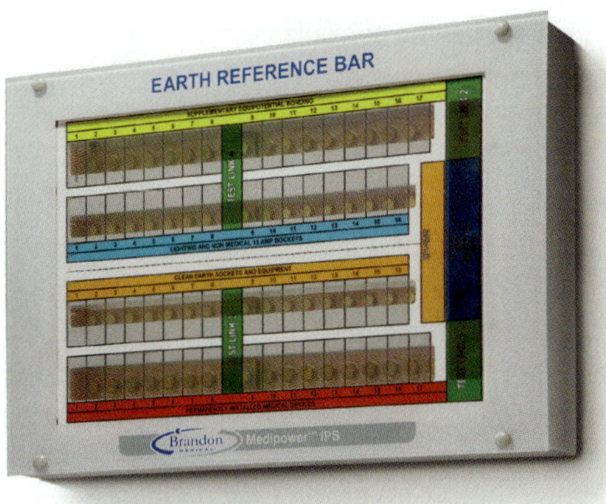

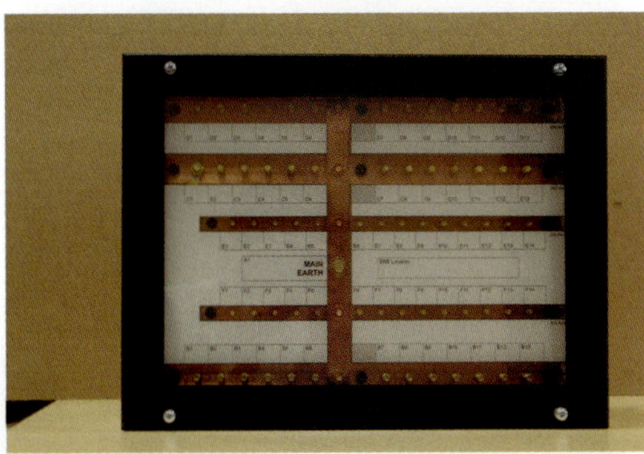

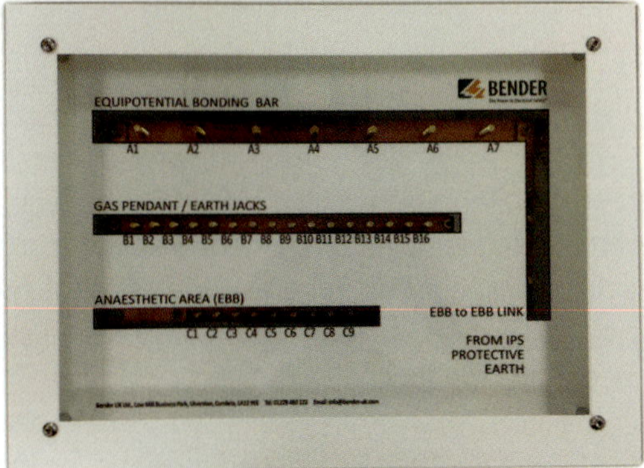

▼ **Figure 14.6** Commercially available equipotential bonding busbars (EBBs) (images courtesy of Brandon Medical, Bender and Starkstrom)

14.3 Changing the terminology

Historically, MEIGaN created a detailed but onerous methodology to reduce touch voltages in the patient environment. As part of this detailed methodology, a requirement for an earthing terminal arrangement (originally known as an earth reference bar (ERB)) was created. This was the point at which all protective conductors were connected.

Even though the term Equipotential Bonding Busbar (EBB) has been used since 2002, the arrangements described in MEIGaN which was published in 2005 are known as earth reference bars. This terminology has been widely adopted across the UK, and as the term is so widely used, manufacturers have been slow to change the name regardless of the naming of the EBB in Regulation 710.415.2.3.

This product is, at the time of writing, marketed as an ERB. However, it is understood from manufacturers that they are in the process of changing the terminology.

14.4 Supplementary equipotential bonding in Group 2 medical locations

Within Group 2 medical locations, there is the added complexity of the medical IT system. In attempting to resolve this, early publications tried to create an arrangement consisting of both bonding conductors and protective conductors to meet the onerous touch voltage requirements set out in both MEIGaN and (S)HTM documentation.

▼ **Figure 14.7** Typical Group 2 medical location

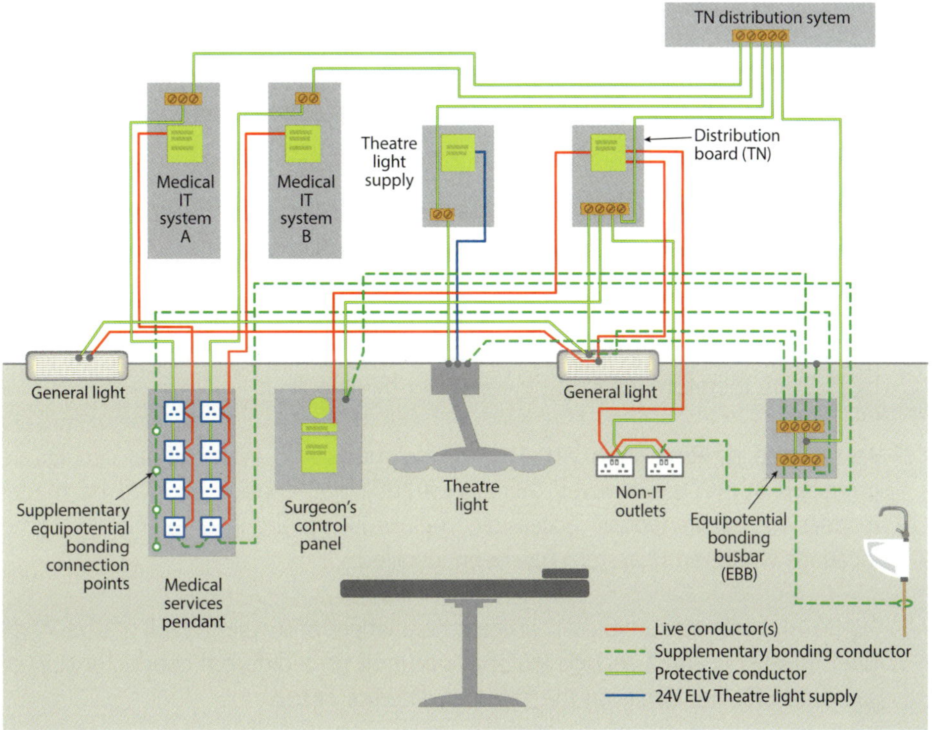

Figure 14.7 is a simplistic representation of the supplementary equipotential bonding arrangement in a typical Group 2 medical location.

As with the Group 1 medical location, the size of the conductors is limited by three factors:

(a) Regulation 544.2.3, which requires a minimum conductor size of 2.5 mm² or 4 mm² if the conductor is unprotected;

(b) the resistance of the exposed-conductive-part to extraneous-conductive-part as suggested in Regulation 710.415.2.2, which is to be not greater than 0.2 Ω in a Group 2 location; and

(c) the resulting voltage between simultaneously accessible parts as required by Regulation 710.411.3.2.5, which is 25 V AC or 60 V DC.

As with the Group 1 medical location, in this instance, even though a maximum value of 0.2 Ω is required by Regulation 710.415.2.2, this is not a performance criterion and there is still a requirement to satisfy touch voltage requirements of Regulation 710.411.3.2.5. This limits the touch voltage (UL) on simultaneously accessible parts to 25 V AC or 60 V DC, which is a performance criterion.

In order to check this criterion has been met, the following formula will need to be applied:

For AC systems:

$$R_A \times I_a \leq 25 \text{ V}$$

Where:

R_A is the sum of the resistance in Ω of the earth electrode and protective conductor for the exposed-conductive-parts.

I_a is the fault current in A of the first fault of negligible impedance between a line conductor and an exposed-conductive-part. The value of I_a takes account of leakage currents and the total earthing impedance of the electrical installation.

In Group 2 medical locations, the requirements for TN circuits to have RCD protection in line with Regulation 415.1.1 still applies ($I_{\Delta n}$ of 30 mA).

As can be seen from the Group 1 calculations, due to the small amount of current flow required to earth to cause disconnection of the faulty circuit those circuits protected by RCD are therefore going to be compliant by default.

As required by Regulation 710.411.3.3, the medical IT system final circuits are not protected by RCDs. However, there is an additional consideration to be made with respect to simultaneously accessible metalwork in Group 2 or Group 1 medical locations where an IT system has been installed.

Figure 14.8 indicates a typical IT arrangement where one system fault has been ignored (indicatively L1) and a second fault has occurred on a different conductor (L2) on the same transformer either on the same or different circuit.

▼ **Figure 14.8** Example of an earth fault path between the exposed-conductive-parts

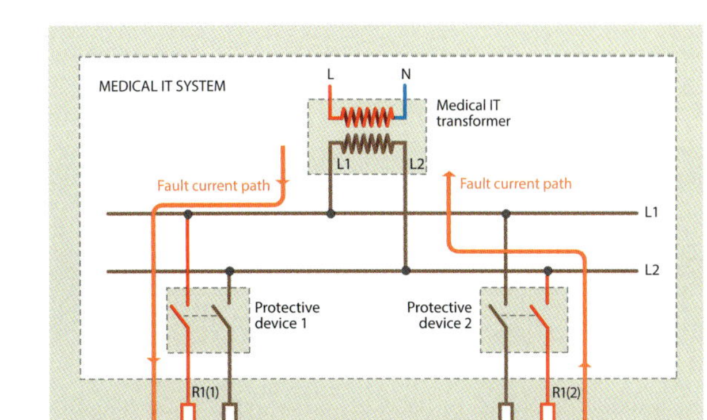

In the above scenario the earth fault path is indicated between the exposed-conductive-parts of each circuit with the path being formed by a combination of the circuit protective conductors associated with the circuit and the supplementary equipotential bonding conductors, which is indicated as the earth fault path on the above diagram.

In order to determine the maximum voltage that could exist between exposed-conductive-parts and extraneous-conductive-parts it is necessary to determine the fault current required to operate the protective device.

▼ **Figure 14.9** Resulting voltage on conductive parts

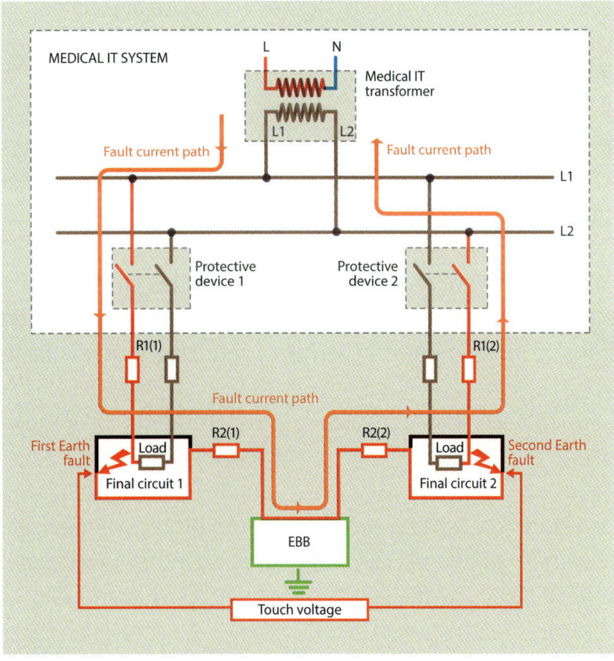

Note: Historically, medical IT system final circuits have been designed with 20 A Type B MCBs.

Below is an extract of Table 2 from BS EN 60898-1:2003+A13:2012 relating to the different values of instantaneous tripping current for the standard types of over protective devices.

▼ **Table 14.3**   Extract of Table 2 from BS EN 60898-1:2003+A13:2012

Type	Range
B	Above 3 I_n up to and including 5 I_n
C	Above 5 I_n up to and including 10 I_n
D	Above 10 I_n up to and including 20 I_n

Consequently, initially applying I_a for the 20 A Type B device from the manufacturer's data would be 100 A (based on 5 I_n).

Thus:

$$0.2 \times 100 = 20 \text{ V}$$

A value of 20 V is acceptable.

However, when applying this to a 20 A Type C device, the maximum value of I_a would be 200 A (10 I_n):

$$0.2 \times 200 = 40 \text{ V}$$

This is not acceptable, and we therefore need to determine a value to meet the requirement. Therefore, by rearranging the formula we can calculate the maximum impedance to maintain the voltage between conductive parts.

$$R_A = 25 \text{ V}/200 = 0.125 \text{ } \Omega$$

Likewise for a Type D with I_a being 400 A, the value would be:

$$R_A = 25 \text{ V}/200 = 0.0625 \text{ } \Omega$$

As this demonstrates, the standard values indicated in early guidance (MEIGaN Annex 1 – now withdrawn, and HTM 06-01) are provided for pre-determined protective device solutions.

Using the above information, where a design varies from a 20 A Type B protective device, the practice of providing separate protective conductors and isolation washers appears almost counterintuitive in terms of reducing touch voltages (U_L).

Designers are to take into account the requirements of Regulation 533.2.1 which states:

The rated current (or current setting) of the protective device shall be chosen in accordance with Regulation 433.1... In certain cases, to avoid unintentional operation, the peak current values of the loads may have to be taken into consideration...

This requirement includes inrush currents etc. In taking this into account, the characteristics of protective devices may be required to be changed from the 20 A Type B devices implied in guidance such as HTM 06-01A. In those instances account should be taken of the resulting touch voltage U_L, which is potentially created by using standard impedance values.

14.5 Other configurations

There are other configurations that will meet the supplementary equipotential bonding requirements of Regulation 710.415.2.1. Topologies indicated in various publications include the protective conductor arrangement within the EBB. In such an instance, the conductor connecting the EBB to the earthing terminal of the local distribution must be sized to accommodate fault current and must also serve as an equipotential bonding conductor.

Other configurations show separate circuit protective conductors to IT systems being joined together at, or adjacent to, the medical IT earthing terminal.

▼ **Figure 14.10** Typical theatre layout

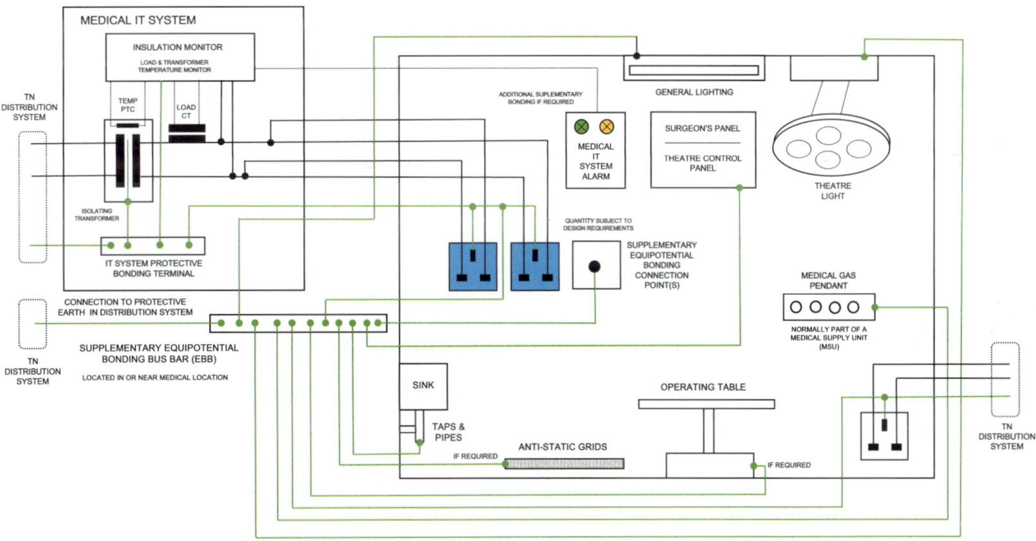

Although there is not one particular method of achieving compliance, the chosen method must satisfy the criteria set out in Regulations 710.415.2.1, 710.411.3.2.5 and 544.2.3.

14.6 Supplementary equipotential bonding connection points

Regulation 710.415.2.1 requires Groups 1 and 2 medical locations to have supplementary equipotential bonding connection points installed. This requirement is to enable the use, if required, of equipotential bonding that leads between the ME equipment and the electrical installation earth connections.

The fitting of these supplementary equipotential bonding connections to ME equipment is not compulsory, according to BS EN 60601-1, as equipotential bonding points are not provided within all medical locations worldwide. Also, BS EN 60601-1 does not specify any dimensions for this connection point other than the marking label to be used as shown in Figure 14.11.

▼ **Figure 14.11** IEC 60617-5021 equipotential symbol

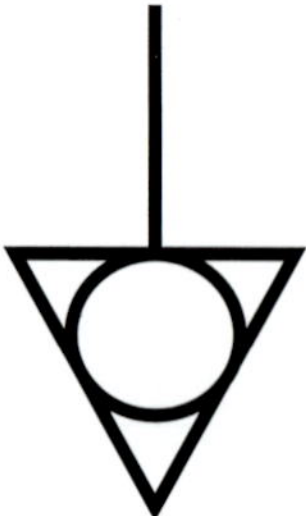

Over time the de-facto standard for the equipotential bonding points has become the German DIN 42801, and is now used almost exclusively on ME equipment that requires such a connection. The connection point mounted on the medical device and electrical installation is a male pin as shown below.

▼ **Figure 14.12** Equipotential bonding pin (male), face plate or trunking mounted (image courtesy of Brandon Medical)

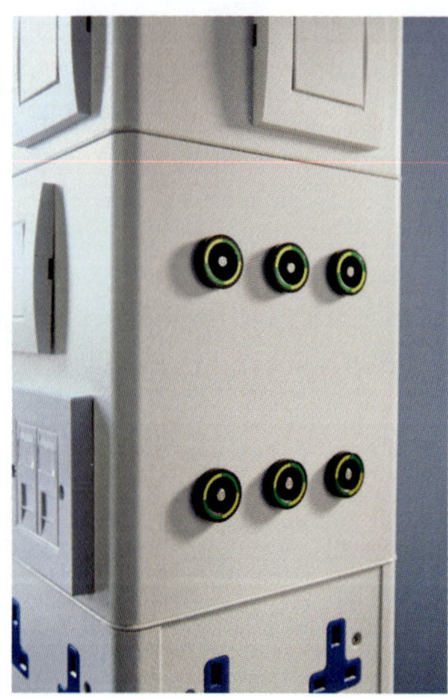

A typical equipotential bonding lead, which consists of a female socket at both ends, is shown below.

▼ **Figure 14.13** Equipotential bonding connection lead (female) (images courtesy of Brandon Medical)

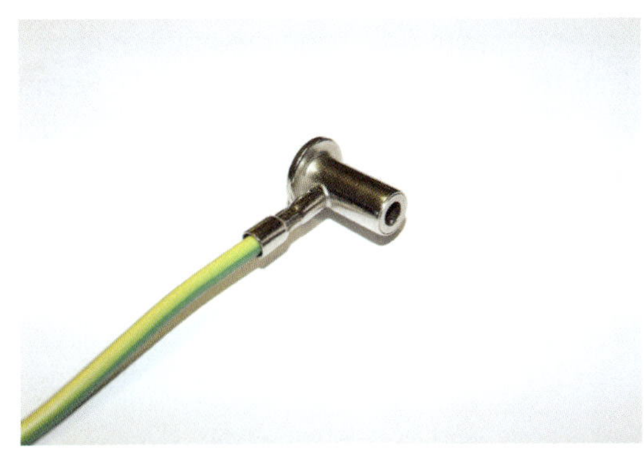

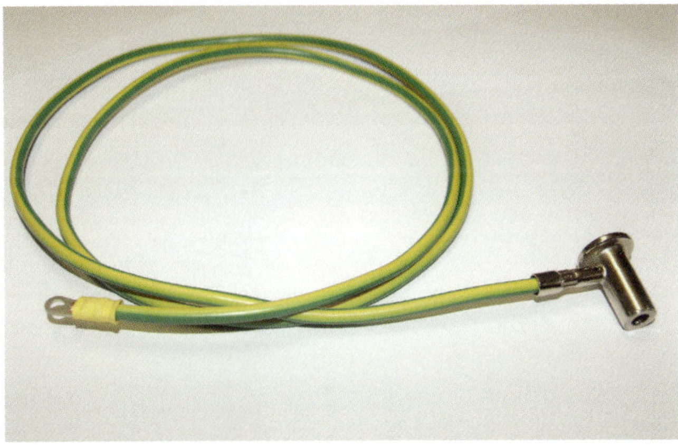

The theory behind the purpose of this equipment is that the use of these equipotential bonding leads can be useful to ensure additional safety should the main ME equipment protective earth become damaged (open circuit) or to ensure excessive touch leakage and contact voltages do not occur between multiple medical devices. Equipotential bonding leads would theoretically be useful when high current equipment, such as mobile X-ray units, are used.

Despite the theories these items are possibly the least used piece of equipment supplied in hospitals; currently, the standard practice is for these to remain unused. It therefore leads to the question of whether they are of any value in the UK, given the UK's reliable earthing and bonding arrangements.

There are those who suggest that these connection leads should be installed as a matter of course and will serve to increase safety, however, this 'blanket' application of the additional supplementary equipotential bonding may give rise to equipment, such as Class II equipment, being unnecessarily bonded to the protective conductors. This incorrect connection of such equipment means, at best, that the equipment is outside its manufacturer's equipment parameters and may not comply with the requirements of BS EN 60601.

This blanket application would therefore require clinical staff to make electrical considerations that are neither within their skill sets or appropriate at the time of a procedure.

To date, much controversy exists as to whether there should be a mandatory number of supplementary equipotential bonding connection points or whether it should be the designer/client/end user to determine the number of points. However, Regulation 710.415.2.1 is clear. The working group responsible for Section 710 are due to review the status of the additional supplementary equipotential bonding connection points during the next phase in the development and updating of IEC 60364-7-710, which may have an effect on future editions of BS 7671.

Medical location lighting

In Groups 1 and 2 medical locations, Regulation 710.559 requires that:

(a) luminaires and lighting circuits to be two different sources of supply; and

(b) one of the supplies should be connected to the electrical supply system for safety services.

This provision provides a level of resilience so that an area remains functional even though it may be at slightly reduced capacity.

This means that, as a general principle, generator-backed supplies should be used throughout. However, this does not preclude the use of other forms of supplies that are considered acceptable, for example, battery inverter units, provided there is a clear understanding of how long the supply is to be maintained by the safety supply.

Whilst other equipment is considered, the preferred alternative supply source is usually a generator because, as long as it is adequately rated and provided with fuel, the supply is considered to be continuous.

15.1 Safety lighting

Standby lighting is defined in BS 5266 as that part of emergency lighting provided to enable normal activities to continue substantially unchanged.

Unlike standby lighting, there is no definition for safety lighting in BS 7671 2008+A3:2015, however, the increase in scope of BS 5266:2016 has introduced a definition for emergency safety lighting as being: "that part of emergency lighting that provides illumination for the safety of people staying in a premise when the supply to the normal lighting fails".

It is apparent from the requirements of Regulation 710.560.9.1 that such lighting refers loosely to emergency lighting. The requirements for emergency lighting stipulate that in the event of mains power failure, the changeover period to the safety services source shall not exceed 15 s. The necessary minimum illuminance shall be provided for the following:

(a) emergency lighting and exit signs;

(b) locations for switchgear and controlgear for emergency generating sets, for main distribution boards of the normal power supply and for power supply for safety services;

(c) rooms in which essential services are intended; in each such room at least one luminaire shall be supplied from the power source for safety services;

(d) locations of central fire alarm and monitoring systems;

(e) rooms of Group 1 medical locations; in each such room at least one luminaire shall be supplied from the power supply source for safety services; and

(f) rooms of Group 2 medical locations: a minimum of 90 % of the lighting shall be supplied from the power source for safety services.

Regulation 710.56 states: 'A power supply for safety services is required which will maintain the supply for continuous operation for a defined period within a pre-set changeover time...'.

As a safety service is defined as ' An electrical system for electrical equipment provided to protect or warn persons in the event of a hazard, or essential to their evacuation from a location'. The requirement for Group 1 and 2 lighting to be connected to a supply for safety services needs full consideration, which means that the requirements of Chapter 56 will apply as well as the specific requirements set out in Section 710.

Chapter 56 includes a number of requirements, one of which is for wiring systems for circuits of safety services being required to be able to operate in fire conditions. This requirement will bring about the need for careful consideration of selection and routing of wiring systems etc.

HTM 06-01(2007) refers to standby lighting making the statement in clause 16.81 that it considers this form of lighting to be a secondary form of emergency lighting, as indicated in BS 5266. As standby lighting will not be available in the reinstatement times required by BS 5266 it cannot be considered an alternative for escape lighting.

Examining the specific requirements for Groups 1 and 2 medical locations, Regulation 710.560.9.1 states: "the luminaires of escape routes shall be arranged on alternate circuits."

These requirements, particularly (e) and (f), are not too dissimilar to those requirements set out in HTM 06-01(2007) for either category B standby lighting or category A respectively.

However, the split between category A and B areas is not always the same as the constraints between Groups 1 and 2 medical locations. In other words, there can be category A standby lighting required in Group 1 medical locations as well as in category B. However, it is unlikely that there are any category B standby systems that are required in a Group 2 medical location due to its use.

It can be seen that the safety services supply does not have to be a non-break supply; it is acceptable for a safety service to maintain a supply for a defined period of time following a pre-set changeover, which, in this instance, is a period not exceeding 15 s – this is the usual start-up time for a generator-backed supply. However, in certain areas, designers may consider the use of inverters and central back up batteries to provide a no-break lighting facility.

Additionally, to keep in line with the requirement for two supplies, it is usual to interleave the lighting circuits not just with a safety and standard supply. Where there are not two separate sources of supply available, provided the supply is connected to an electrical safety source consideration with an appropriate risk assessment may be given to multiple final circuits from the same distribution board. This arrangement provides added resilience over a single final circuit which would be not compliant with the requirements of BS 7671.

There is also a requirement for lighting circuits on escape routes to be configured so that alternative lights are on different circuits. Healthcare premises that use progressive horizontal evacuation (PHE), alternative routes through wards etc. should be subject to the same considerations.

The question of how we define a medical location is often raised when looking at different healthcare schemes.

When designing a medical location in accordance with Section 710 of BS 7671 the following procedure is recommended as a minimum requirement:

(a) engage clinical staff to determine individual/specific room use and procedures carried out;
(b) ascertain the type of applied parts in use in the room;
(c) consider the threat to life and safety through discontinuity of supply; and
(d) refer to informative Table A710 as necessary to support the process.

Once Table A710 has been consulted:

(a) check with the clinicians that they will not be changing the use at a later date, which may require re-classification of the medical location; and
(b) confirm the power requirements of any special equipment, for example, X-ray equipment may require very low line impedance (not referring to Z_s).

In order to be successful, the process should have a level of engagement with the appropriate clinical service providers to determine room usage and the potential for the room to be used for other procedures which may have a more onerous requirement that its room name suggests.

Upon satisfactory completion of the process, the results should be agreed with all stakeholders and recorded as a design statement/reference point. This will allow successive reviews to appreciate considerations made at particular design stage.

This process described is relatively straightforward, however, to avoid errors it should be noted that, just as engineers are not necessarily aware of all the implications of clinical procedures, likewise clinicians may not be aware of the electro-technical aspects of the selection process when determining a location.

Therefore to avoid disappointment or potential conflict; a clear understanding of what is required and what is being provided is essential at design, construction and commissioning stage.

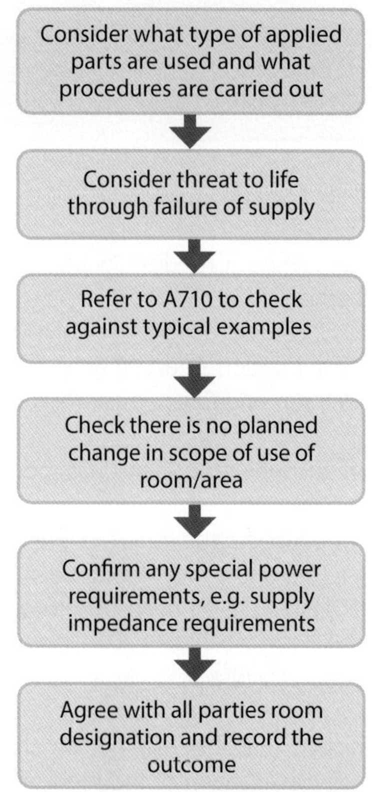

Figure 16.1 is a suggested flowchart for discussion with clinical staff. At each point this chart expects that the designer would provide clear and simple explanation of the impact of each decision.

Group 0 design considerations

This is, according to BS 7671, the lowest categorization of any of the medical locations. In these rooms there are very few restrictions/requirements over and above those that are set out in the general requirements of BS 7671.

Group 0 medical locations are rooms and areas where no applied parts are intended to be used and where discontinuity (failure) of the supply cannot cause danger to life.

▼ **Figure 17.1** Example of a Group 0 medical location (image courtesy of Brandon Medical)

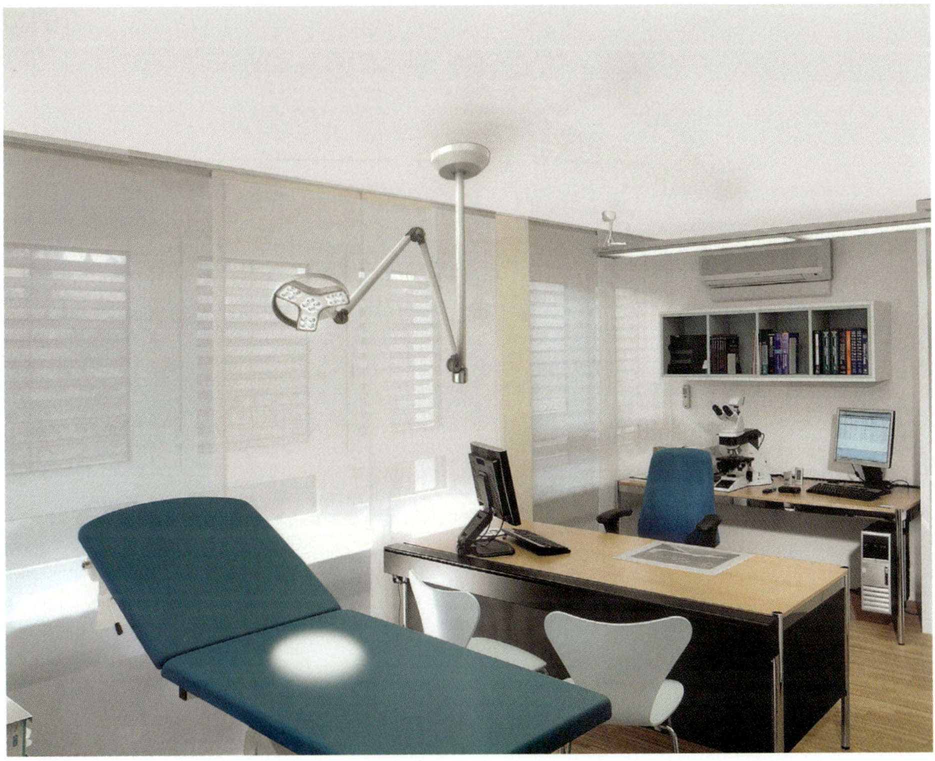

This will apply to the majority of the hospital areas such as patient waiting and circulation areas, as well as:

(a) consultant examination rooms;
(b) consenting rooms; and
(c) massage rooms.

In these locations many but not all of the specific requirements of Section 710 are relaxed, however, this area is part of a healthcare facility so will have functions and services that are integral to lighting that would not normally be found in an office environment, such as generator-backed lighting to give continuity of service after the failure of electricity, etc.

Whilst there may be nothing particularly special about a Group 0 medical location in terms of disconnection times, etc., it is important to remember that it is usually part of a healthcare premises and as such contains consulting/consenting rooms, nursing stations, touch down bases along with ancillary services etc. all of which form part of the overall patient experience.

In addition, it may be unrealistic to allow the parameters to be different, for example, disconnection times, etc., as the Group 0 medical location is located or, as more appropriately termed, 'embedded', within a series of higher rated rooms and locations.

As such, in relaxing any requirement to a Group 0 medical location, the overall impact of such a relaxation should be considered.

Group 1 design considerations

BS 7671 defines a Group 1 medical location as:

Medical location where discontinuity (failure) of the electrical supply does not represent a threat to the safety of the patient and applied parts are intended to be used:

- *externally*
- *invasively to any part of the body except where Group 2 applies.*

▼ **Figure 18.1** Example of a Group 1 medical location (image courtesy of IBI Group)

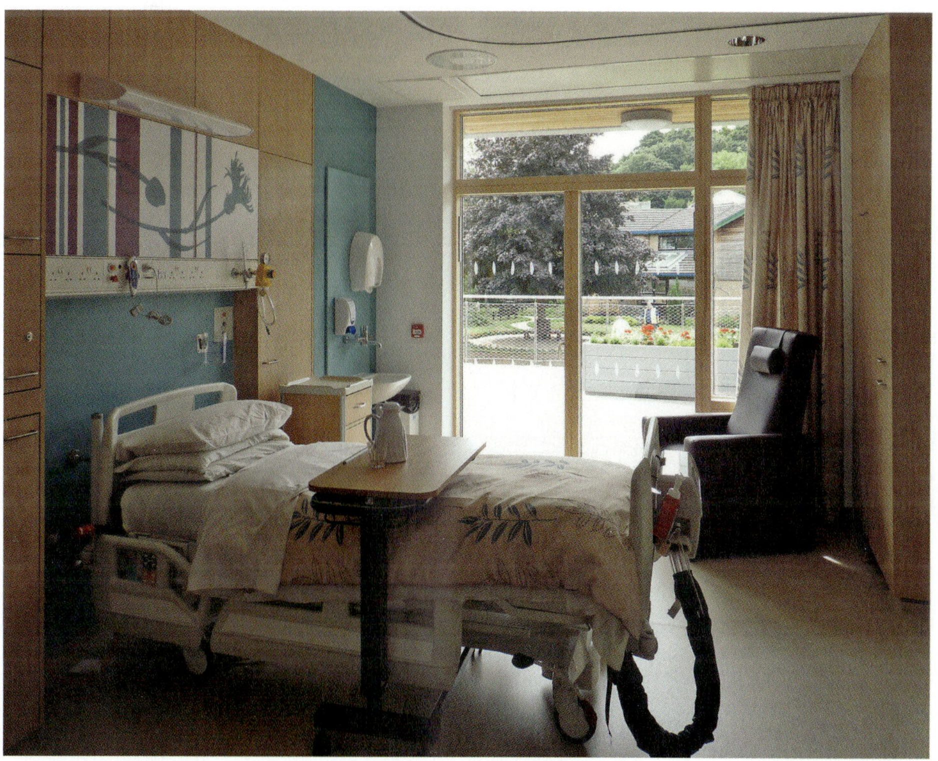

As part of the process of designing a medical location it is assumed that the recommended processes indicated in previous sections have been followed in order to determine the group rating of the particular location. This is set out in the flow chart of Figure 18.2.

▼ **Figure 18.2** Liaison with clinicians

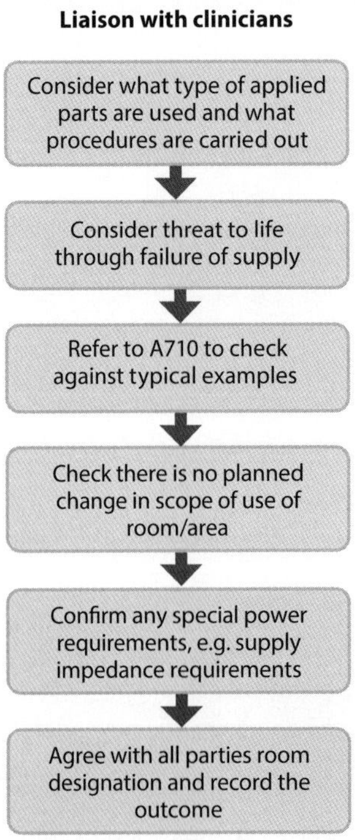

Once determined it is important to consider the individual factors affecting any design, including:

1 reduced disconnection times;
2 reduced touch voltage (25 V);
3 safety circuit design;
4 requirements for RCD protection of TN circuits up to 63 A; and
5 additional protection using supplementary equipotential bonding.

18.1 Maximum disconnection times

The maximum disconnection times for a Group 1 or Group 2 medical location are more onerous than those of the general requirements of BS 7671.

▼ **Table 18.1** Extracted from Table 710 (BS 7671)

System	$25\,V < U_0 \leq 50\,V$ (seconds)		$50\,V < U_0 \leq 120\,V$ (seconds)		$120\,V < U_0 \leq 230\,V$ (seconds)		$230\,V < U_0 \leq 400\,V$ (seconds)		$U_0 > 400\,V$ (seconds)	
	AC	DC	AC	DC	AC	DC	AC	DC	AC	DC
TN	5	5	0.3	2	0.3	0.5	0.05	0.06	0.02	0.02
TT	5	5	0.15	0.2	0.05	0.1	0.02	0.06	0.02	0.02

Note: In TN systems, a value of 25 V AC or 60 V DC may be met with protective equipotential bonding if it complies with the disconnection time in accordance with Table 710.

Typically, values for TN and TT systems are reduced to 0.3 s and 0.05 s respectively. However, the note below Table 710 does not refer to the 'not to be exceeded' values in Regulation 710.415.2.2.

18.2 Supplementary equipotential bonding: Group 1 medical locations

▼ **Figure 18.3** Group 1 location supplemental bonding arrangement

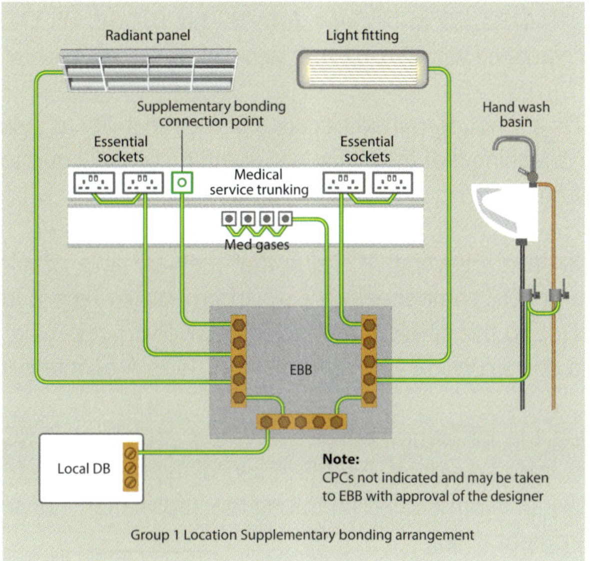

In order to meet the requirements of Regulation 710.415.2.2, and to limit the voltage presented between simultaneously accessible exposed or extraneous-conductive-parts in accordance with Regulation 710.411.3.2.5, supplementary equipotential bonding is to be applied to the installation. As the requirement in Regulation 710.415.2.2 relates to parts that may not be simultaneously accessible, i.e. any socket-outlet terminal, the bonding should be applied so as to achieve the requirement which is not just simultaneously accessible conductive parts.

The supplementary equipotential bonding conductors are also required to meet the requirements of Regulation 544.2.3.

▼ **Figure 18.4** Typical ward – bed area

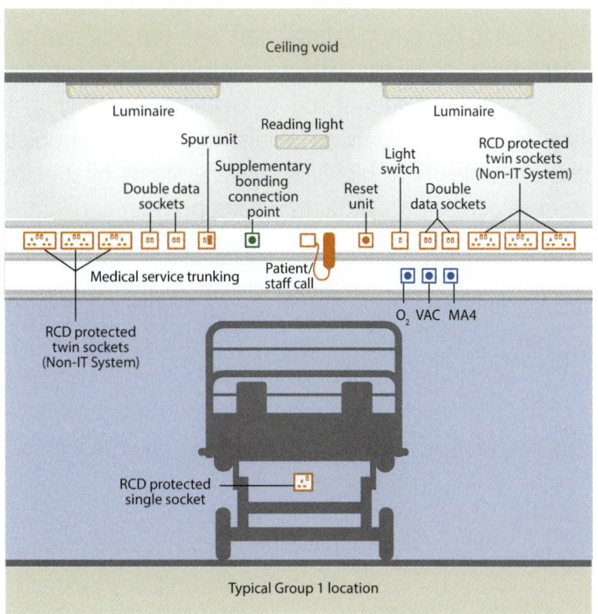

In Group 1 medical locations, a maximum value of 0.7 Ω is stated, however, this is a maximum value and must be considered in conjunction with the requirements for 0.3 s disconnection times and the limiting touch voltage of 25 V AC and 60 V DC under fault conditions.

18.3 Use of RCDS

In Group 1 medical locations, all TN final circuits that have a protective device rated at 63 A or less are required to be RCD protected. These RCDs are required by Regulation 710.411.3.2.5 to be Type A to BS EN 61008, BS EN 61009 or potentially Type B in accordance with IEC 62423, depending on the type of fault current.

Type AC RCDs are not permitted because of their inability to detect DC component in a waveform, meaning that they may not operate correctly due to the presence of DC in the waveform.

Type A RCDs have a limiting DC value that they are able to tolerate, which is in the order of 6 mA of DC component on a waveform, whilst Type B RCDs will operate with DC signals. Due to the different technologies involved, the Type B RCD is less readily available and costs considerably more than its Type A counterpart.

In highlighting the difference between Type A and Type B RCDs, this Guide does not advocate the omission of Type B in lieu of Type A; instead, it advocates that the designer make an informed decision using the information available, including the load and the equipment types.

18.4 Operation of RCDs

Where RCDs are used it is essential to consider the effects that an RCD tripping may have on patient safety. This means ensuring that there are an adequate number of individually protected circuits available in any given area to take account of the total expected equipment leakage currents and the effect a faulty appliance may have on other connected equipment. For example, in a haemodialysis unit, it would be advisable to protect each haemodialysis machine supply with its own individual RCD and provide additional RCD protected circuits for other mains equipment.

18.5 Difficult to define locations

The final decision as to the group rating is left with the designer to justify in conjunction with the relevant levels of liaison with the clinician/end users/client teams. This Guide deals with the process of identifying a location and highlighting areas that have been identified as being contentious. Whilst the list of examples in this Guide is not exhaustive, the examples here highlight considerations of specific risks and perceived hazards in order to achieve a satisfactory solution.

Other types of medical care 19

19.1 Mental health units

These types of units are often misunderstood, particularly by those professionals that claim a level of expertise in their design and construction.

In terms of this type of unit, they are often classified as a Group 0 medical location installation. Whilst this Guide does not support pre-determined decisions about group ratings, mental health units have their own separate challenges, which designers must overcome.

Typical mental health units consist of individual rooms or, in some instances (which are becoming fewer and fewer) dormitories where patients have their own space or area. Unlike many other units patients can be admitted for weeks and months, often against their will.

The general requirements for the electrical installation in a mental health unit is about removing any additional risk that electrical equipment, including fixed electrical equipment, can present to patients and staff in certain conditions, without, as far as practicable, making the installation institutionalized or prison-like.

19.1.1 Electrical equipment

In order to reduce the likelihood of injury from electricity, the electrical installation is normally quite robust with much of the installation designed to avoid contact with the patient wherever possible.

Historically, even before the virtual autonomic use of RCDs in the general requirements of BS 7671 became the norm, RCDs were required by the Health Building Note HBN 35 *Accommodation for people with mental illness* (this has since been superseded by HBN 03-01: *Adult Acute Mental Health Units*).

The RCD is a useful piece of additional protection, particularly given that patients in such units through illness, may wish to harm themselves or, through their behaviour, cause damage to property. As a consequence of this damage this may create a situation that may give rise to danger to themselves or others.

19.1.2 Specialist treatment areas within mental health units

Generally, treatments undertaken within mental health units include various types of therapy. This therapy does not often use the same level of ME equipment that may be seen on a medical or surgical ward.

Having a mental illness does not exempt a patient from requiring other medical interventions and it is now recognised that a patient's physical well-being can have a positive effect on their mental health.

Specialist diagnostics will be carried out in the relevant diagnostic department of a hospital. Additionally, there will be other procedures and observations that will be carried out by the mental health nurses, either in treatment rooms on wards or in patient bedrooms. Examples of these would be ECGs, etc.

▼ **Figure 19.1** Medical equipment in use

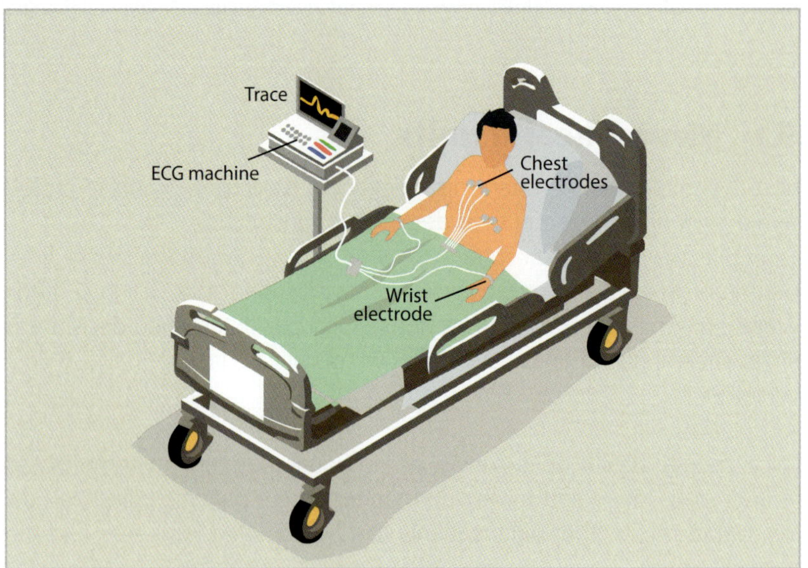

Applying the logic of Table A710, a patient bedroom and a treatment room on a mental health unit may therefore be considered a Group 1 location.

There would be obvious differences between a mental health unit bed space and a general hospital bed space. One such difference is the requirement for supplementary equipotential bonding points. These connection points are generally unused in medical and surgical applications. Therefore, it would be inadvisable to encourage the use of supplementary equipotential bonding connection points and their leads in the environments, as such leads could be considered a potential hazard if left or lost on the unit.

▼ **Figure 19.2** Typical equipotential connection lead (image courtesy of Brandon Medical)

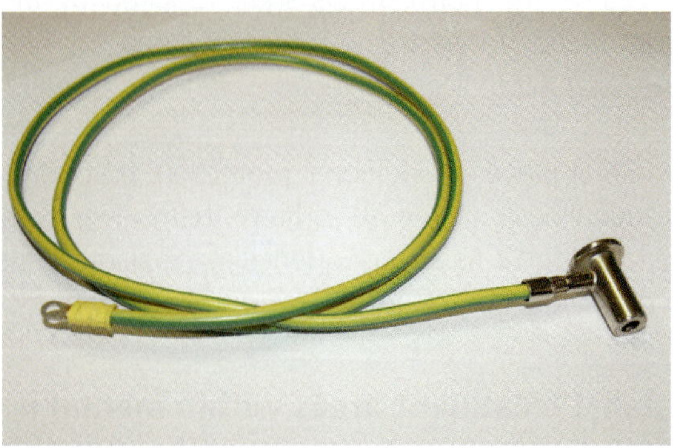

This may be in conflict with Regulation 710.415.2.1 of BS 7671, however, it is the responsibility of the designer to consider the risks involved in the positioning of equipment. In this instance, it may well be more appropriate to cover any difference in requirements with a risk assessment that is agreed with clinicians and is used as a design statement. It may be necessary to record this on the Electrical Installation Certificate as an agreed departure under Regulation 120.3.

In addition to bedrooms and treatment rooms, there are other specialist procedures carried out in specialist treatment suites within mental health units, such as electro-convulsive therapy (ECT). This involves applied parts being attached to the patient to apply a charge of electricity that induces a convulsion as part of a therapeutic intervention.

The areas in which such treatments are undertaken should be treated as at least Group 1 medical locations, even though the patient may be anaesthetised, there are generally no intubation procedures carried out and, as such, mechanical ventilators are not used for this brief intervention. However, this is another area that will require detailed discussion with the clinicians and the outcome of which should be assessed and covered in a risk assessment and consequent design statement.

The fundamental elements for safety are to ensure that robust and fit-for-purpose equipment is selected, ligature points are avoided and, where necessary, security fixings are used to prevent unwanted tampering.

19.2 Haemodialysis

The area in which haemodialysis is undertaken has, since the publication of IEC 60364-7-710 2002, been classified as a Group 1 medical location.

19.2.1 Haemodialysis classification logic

Haemodialysis is carried out in different formats across the UK. It is understood that some can be carried out in the home, whereas the majority of dialysis interventions take place either in hospital or specialist satellite units.

In hospitals, there is usually no problem with achieving the requirements of a Group 1 medical location. The requirements are set out in informative Annex A710 of BS 7671.

▼ **Figure 19.3** Extract from Table A710

17 Intensive care room			X	X[a]	X
18 Angiographic examination room			X	X[a]	X
19 Haemodialysis room		X			X
20 Magnetic resonance imaging (MRI) room		X	X	X	X
21 Nuclear medicine		X			X
22 Premature baby room			X	X[a]	X
23 Intermediate Care Unit (IMCU)			X	X	X
a Luminaires and life-support medical electrical equipment which needs power supply within 0.5s or or less. b Not being an operating theatre.					

There are occasionally issues in achieving full Group 1 medical location compliance when using satellite dialysis installations that are remote from the main services of a hospital, and that do not have the benefit of available back-up generators. In instances such as these the designer will be required to mitigate this by other means.

In Group 1 medical locations, the preferred method of providing a safety source is usually focused around the use of back-up generators, as this gives a long-term supply that is comparable to, but not as reliable as, the mains supply. However, the requirement is for a connection to a safety service and must meet the requirements of BS 7671.

These requirements can be dealt with in a number of ways, including the provision of other facilities and services to meet the safety services requirements. As these may be time restricted by, for example, the discharge of UPS batteries, a design statement/risk assessment will be required so that all persons operating the satellite facility understand how a loss in mains supply affects the operation of the unit and what the building operators (usually the clinicians) need to do in the event of loss of mains power. For example, the unit would have to be closed immediately if there is no reverse osmosis (RO) water (a form of purified water supply used in dialysis) being processed to the equipment, or, in the case where a standard water supply is on a boosted cold water main, no water in the WCs, preventing adequate sanitation.

19.2.2 Dialysis process

In the UK there are a number of different dialysis procedures; most of them involve connection through access points (fistulas) in the arm or leg as indicated below.

▼ **Figure 19.4** Typical dialysis arrangement

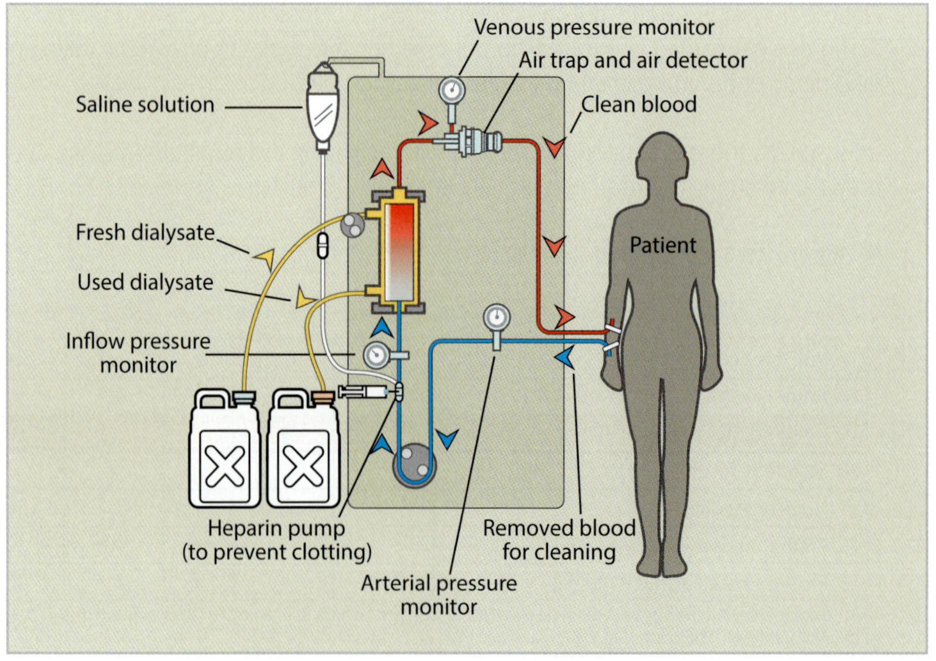

19.2.3 CVC dialysis

In addition to this method and peritoneal dialysis, a form of dialysis that has raised concerns with engineers has been central venous catheter dialysis (CVC dialysis). This involves the provision of a catheter inserted into the heart. This is indicated diagrammatically in Figure 19.5 along with a picture of how the catheter connection would look.

▼ **Figure 19.5** Catheter connection

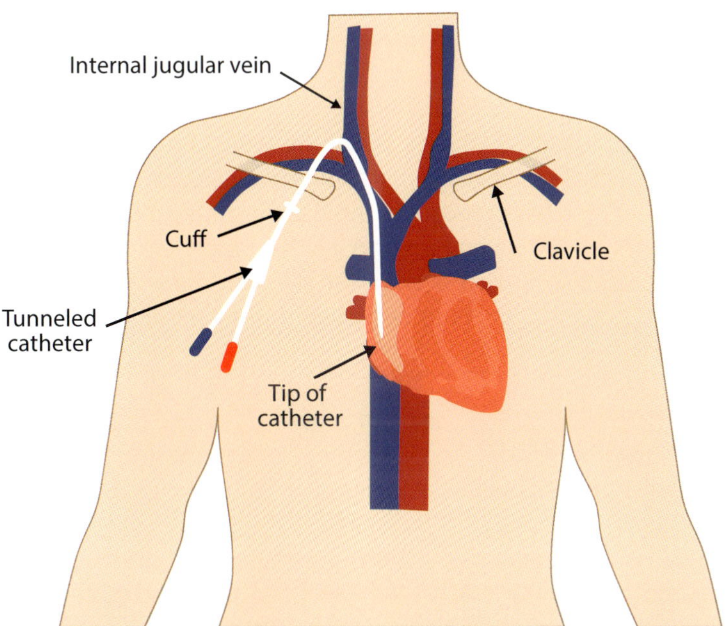

This direct entry method has a number of risks associated with it, however, anecdotal information from clinical professionals suggests that the risk to these patients is infection rather than electrocution through 'alleged' microshock or loss of power during the procedure. These risks are dealt with by the clinical teams and healthcare professionals – usually by having the patient change their behaviours and employ strict hygiene when handling the catheter.

Typically, this type of procedure has automatically classified a location as being Group 2 due to the intracardiac procedures. The definition of a Group 2 location is as follows:

"Group 2. Medical location where applied parts are intended to be used, and where discontinuity (failure) of the supply can cause danger to life, in applications such as:

- *intracardiac procedures*
- *vital treatments and surgical operations."*

Research into the use of CVC dialysis has revealed that the loss of supply to the machine does not represent a danger to the patient and as such the procedure does not fully meet the definition of a Group 2 location.

Historical guidance, such as MEIGaN Annex 1 (now withdrawn) and other publications that referenced medical device standards without necessarily applying the information within the references standards have led to a misunderstanding relating to ME equipment standards. The concern relates to a misunderstanding about the type of equipment in use. Historically, a number of haemodialysis machines were categorised under IEC 60601 as being BF rated instead of the correct CF rating, over the years this has since been rectified so that all equipment used in intracardiac procedures being CF rated according to IEC/BS EN 60601.

This specific detail should not concern electrical building installation designers as it is the responsibility of the clinician to use the correct equipment in line with the relevant medical device directives.

Referring to published information about the electrical hazards associated with CVC dialysis, it is possible to identify where the misunderstanding originates. The concern relates to Type B and BF applied parts; this equipment has a normal condition maximum leakage current of 100 µA and a single fault condition leakage of 500 µA. This value, if it was to come into contact directly with the heart through, for example, a catheter, could produce enough current to cause ventricular fibrillation (VF), which could cause significant injury or death.

However, if a Type B or BF applied part is used this would mean that the operator had used the wrong equipment. The correct equipment for use with cardiac procedures, heart catheterization or similar activities such as CVC dialysis, is a machine that has been classified as having 'cardiac floating' (CF) applied parts. In other words, it is a piece of ME equipment that meets the requirements of the medical devices directive and is suitably isolated so as to minimize leakage currents to a generally accepted level.

This effectively means that the correct equipment should be used for the procedure being carried out, which is no different than in any other industry, i.e. using the right tool for the job at hand!

▼ **Figure 19.6** Extract from BS EN 60601-1 with CF values of leakage highlighted

Symbol	Applied part type	Definition/description	Normal Condition (NC)	Single Fault Condition (SFC)
	Type B Applied Part	**TYPE B APPLIED PART** APPLIED PART complying with the specified requirements of BS EN 60601 to provide protection against electric shock, particularly regarding allowable PATIENT LEAKAGE CURRENT and PATIENT AUXILIARY CURRENT	100µA	500µA
	Type BF Applied Part	**TYPE BF APPLIED PART** F-TYPE APPLIED PART complying with the specified requirements of BS EN 60601 to provide a higher degree of protection against electric shock than that provided by TYPE B APPLIED PARTS	100µA	500µA
	Type CF Applied Part	**TYPE CF APPLIED PART** F-TYPE APPLIED PART complying with the specified requirements BS EN 60601 to provide a higher degree of protection against electric shock than that provided by TYPE BF APPLIED PARTS	10µA	50µA

The above values are for a.c. current and for a single applied part only. Other values exist for d.c. and multiple applied parts.

The previous concerns were therefore founded on a series of misunderstandings as to how ME equipment is applied into the electrical circuit.

There is a theory amongst some engineers that the use of a medical IT transformer will provide protection against 'microshock'. This is ill thought through as the medical isolation transformer standard allows a leakage current of up to 500 µA (0.5 mA) to flow, which is many times larger than the recommended requirements of BS EN 60601. Further information about myths relating to medical IT supplies is contained in Appendix 2.

Additionally, there is much concern about touch voltages, when in fact the only voltages that a patient can touch directly is the table that they are lying on and other exposed- or extraneous-conductive-parts within reach of them. In an installation that is correctly designed in accordance with BS 7671, even under an enduring fault condition, without RCD protection, the maximum touch voltage between exposed-conductive-parts and extraneous-conductive-parts has to be maintained at 25 V. This is completely different from the voltages and currents that may give rise to ventricular fibrillation detailed in BS EN 60601-1.

A particular concern about touch voltages comes, in part, from the use of haemodialysis equipment with Type B applied parts, since the patient is then effectively connected to earth via the machine connections. If they then touch another conductive part that is at a different potential to the haemodialysis machine a current could flow. If CVC dialysis was being performed with this Type B applied part, any current above 50 µA (50 mV) could be dangerous.

However, within the patient environment only ME equipment meeting Medical Device Regulations 2002 (as amended) should be used. This ensures that there is no source of touch voltage (touch leakage current above 500 µA), even under fault conditions of the ME equipment.

Additionally, with the correct application of BS 7671, the protective supplementary equipotential bonding resistance and the addition of RCD protection will not allow any contact voltages to exceed 25 V before the protective device operates and disconnects the fault.

Maintaining the wiring for the exclusive use of the medical location also ensures that coupling of faults from external sources is limited.

19.3 Potential hazard

One possible source of hazard is when the patient is allowed to use electrical devices while they are undergoing treatment. This may include the use of a laptop computer, music player or mobile phone, often connected to a mains socket for charging and power. This scenario is not as bad as would first seem since most domestic devices that are likely to be used will be Class II. As such, the maximum possible leakage current that could be expected if the patient touches these devices is limited to 250 µA. In other words, even if a medical IT system was installed, no additional benefit would occur since this has a higher maximum leakage than the Class II domestic devices.

The diagram below indicates a typical CVC dialysis arrangement, using a CF applied parts machine, with the entry point in the chest.

There are those who consider that there is a risk of microshock through the equipment to the patient's heart through the connection to earth but this is only possible when the incorrect type of equipment, with B applied parts, is used.

▼ **Figure 19.7** Using CF rated medical equipment

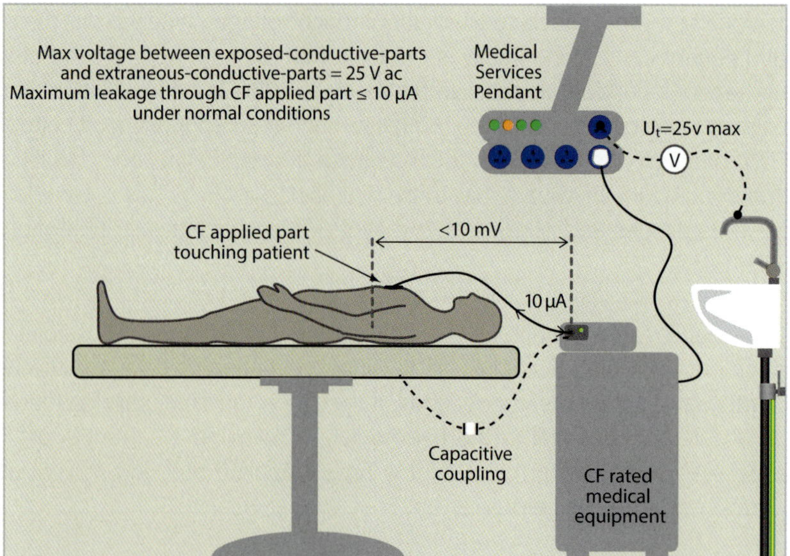

As can be seen in the diagram, the use of the correct ME equipment and a BS 7671 compliant electrical installation means that there is no excessive current flowing and hence no risk to the patient of receiving a 'microshock', even when there is a maximum touch voltage of 25 V AC between an extraneous-conductive-part and an exposed-conductive-parts are present.

19.4 Unrealistic expectations

Previous guidance has concentrated on providing an unrealistic requirement of reducing 'touch voltages' to 10 mV, which equates to 10 μA – which is the standard for CF-rated ME equipment in normal conditions. The thought that an electrical installation with all the different variables in supplies, equipment usage and neighbouring circuits that will affect the installation could meet this expectation is incredibly naive!

An electrical installation cannot meet the rigorous requirements of BS EN 60601 and the Medical Device Directive.

In Figure 19.8, the maximum leakage current passing through the CF applied part via any catheter, etc. is limited to less than 10 µA, due to the onerous requirements of the medical device standards on the equipment.

▼ **Figure 19.8** Indicative block diagram of CF-rated medical equipment

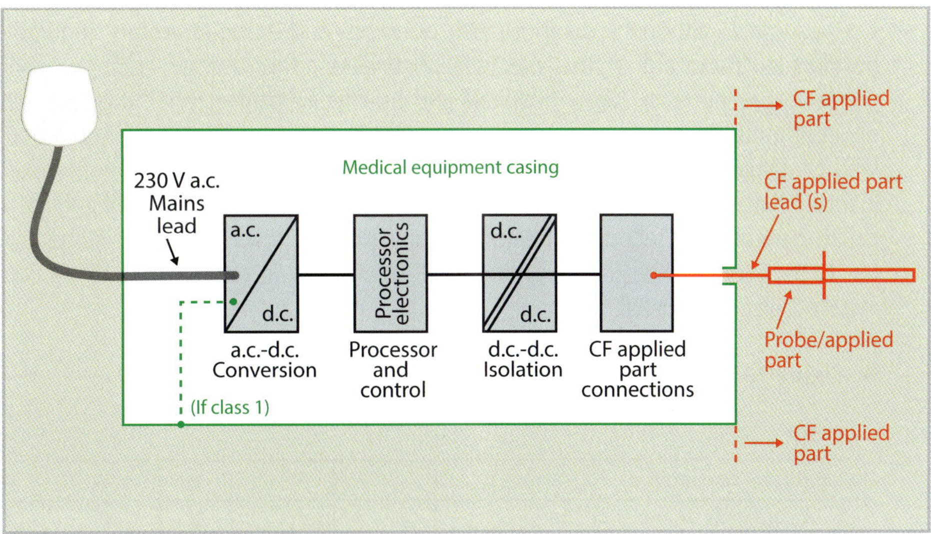

Figure 19.8 provides an understanding of the level of electrical isolation required by a product to achieve the required standard and hence the CF rating. The various stages indicate how there is absolutely no connection between the mains supply, the earthing system and the CF applied part.

Obviously, a similar but less onerous process is provided to BF and Type B applied parts and the ME equipment that the parts are connected to.

As previously stated many misunderstandings have been made due to much of the early haemodialysis equipment being only Type B and BF, hence, under normal conditions, could allow leakage currents to flow though patients that were in excess of the recognised values for CF applications. This would risk ventricular fibrillation in the patient. This danger was often mitigated by following the manufacturer's instructions and ensuring that the patient could not touch any device unless it was CF rated.

These days, equipment should be CF rated or should have been retrofitted with components to give the CF level of protection to allow adequate patient safety for CVC and similar patients.

There are technical papers that suggest solutions using medical IT systems in conjunction with additional supplementary equipotential bonding or for economy just to use supplementary equipotential bonding in order to provide an adequate level of safety.

The arrangement suggested in these papers is questionable as it can be seen that the electrical installation earth should not be connected directly to any applied part that is near to, or in contact with, the heart. Since a medical IT system may serve to minimise earth leakages up to 500 µA, this is still too high to protect the CVC patient if a machine with Type B applied parts was to be inappropriately used. The 500 µA is no different to the equipment leakage current with an open circuit earth, so no additional safety will have been achieved.

In terms of connection of the equipotential bonding connection points, it should be noted that BS EN 60601-1 does not mandate ME equipment to be fitted with equipotential bonding connection points so, regardless of the provision, it may well not be possible to use such equipment due to the medical equipment not requiring or being fitted with a connection facility.

Consequently, although equipotential bonding and supplementary equipotential bonding is important in the electrical installation, the use of additional bonding points is questionable. Many hospitals and healthcare professionals working in these environments do not use the connection points. Using inappropriate equipment can lead to danger for the patient, regardless of the level of local bonding. For example, inappropriate equipment may deliver a leakage current of such a magnitude as to cause danger. The recommendation for any process involving heart catheterization has to therefore be the use of CF-rated ME equipment in conjunction with a correctly installed electrical installation to BS 7671.

▼ **Figure 19.9** Extract from Table A710

17 Intensive care room			X	X[a]	X
18 Angiographic examination room			X	X[a]	X
19 Haemodialysis room	X				X
20 Magnetic resonance imaging (MRI) room	X	X	X	X	
21 Nuclear medicine	X			X	
22 Premature baby room			X	X[a]	X
23 Intermediate Care Unit (IMCU)			X	X	X
a Luminaires and life-support medical electrical equipment which needs power supply within 0.5s or or less. b Not being an operating theatre.					

Despite there being intracardiac procedures in CVC dialysis there is no danger to life through failure of the supply and it is not a life support in line with Regulation 710.560.6.1.1, the suggested Group 1 rating is valid and its positioning in Annex 710 is justified.

Finally, it must be remembered that Annex 710 is a guide only. The designer, in conjunction with the clinical staff, should determine the actual group rating of the room and provide additional or even reduced measures. When varying from the norm it is recommended that a risk assessment and, consequently, design statement is provided, which should be recorded on any certification and will eventually form part of the operation and maintenance manuals.

Group 2 design considerations 20

The focus in most textbooks and literature for Group 2 medical locations primarily focuses on operating theatres and, in particular, intra-cardiac procedures (possibly due to misunderstanding relating to medical electrical equipment ratings) that are carried out in specialist units.

▼ **Figure 20.1** Typical Group 2 location (image courtesy of Brandon Medical)

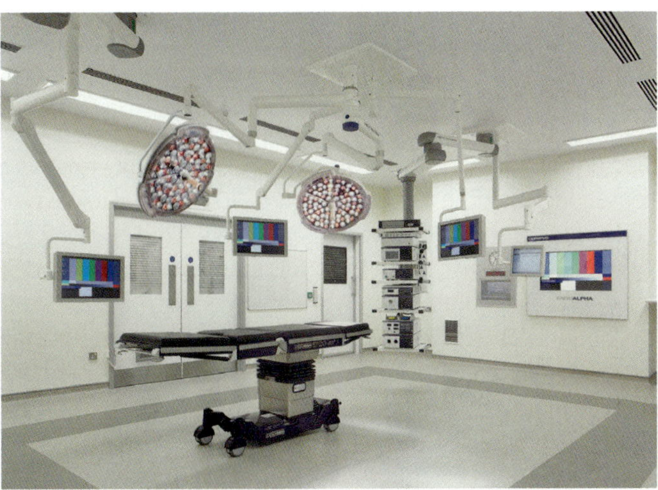

A Group 2 medical location is defined in BS 7671 as follows:

Group 2. *Medical location where applied parts are intended to be used, and where discontinuity (failure) of the supply can cause danger to life, in applications such as:*

- *intracardiac procedures*
- *vital treatments and surgical operations.*

There are a great number of other areas in a hospital that attract less literary attention than the intra-cardiac areas. The patients in other Group 2 locations, such as general surgery, intensive care units or A & E resus areas, are equally in as much need of the special requirements and back-up facilities. Patients in intensive care units, for instance, are normally long-term patients compared with patients undergoing longer, complicated surgical procedures.

▼ **Figure 20.2** Group 2 bed position with wall trunking

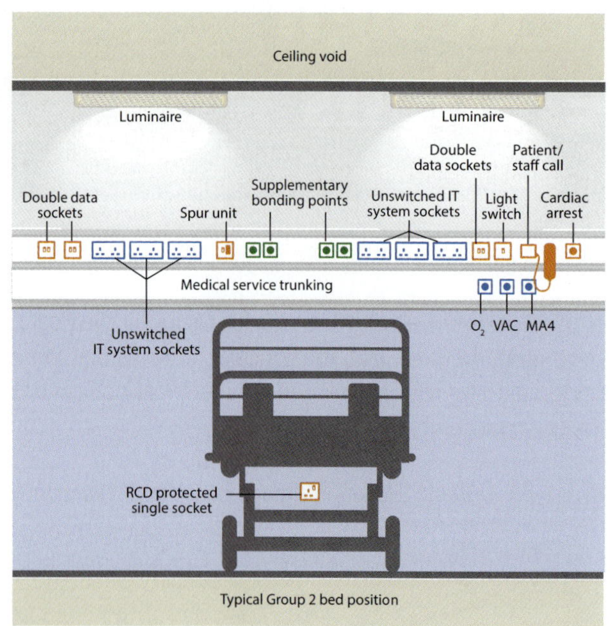

As identified above, Group 2 medical locations do not only exist as operating theatres or catheterisation labs. The layout in Figure 20.2 is that of a typical Group 2 bed location. This may be an intensive care bed, where fixed trunking is used, or it may be a recovery or trauma/resuscitation bed (ME equipment and monitors not indicated).

In multiple bedded Group 2 locations, such as intensive care units, services such as power, gases, etc. are provided on articulated service pendants as indicated in Figure 20.3.

▼ **Figure 20.3** Articulated pendant commonly used in Group 2 locations (Image courtesy of Starkstrom)

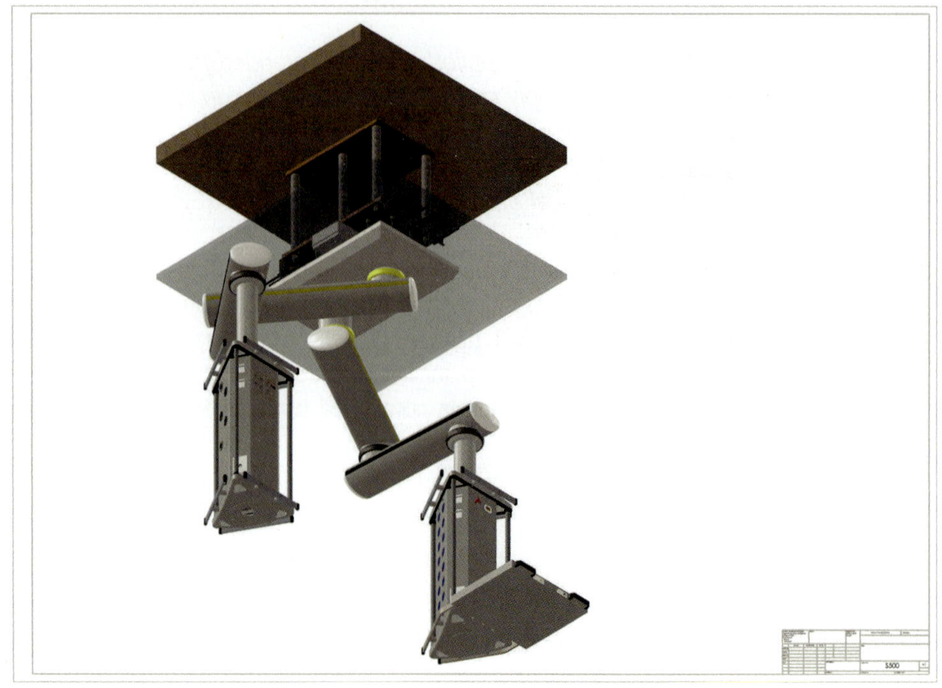

A Guide to Electrical Installations in Medical Locations
© The Institution of Engineering and Technology

In designing any medical location it is assumed that the recommended process indicated in previous sections has been followed to determine the group classification of the particular location, as set out in Figure 20.4.

▼ **Figure 20.4** Liaison with clinicians

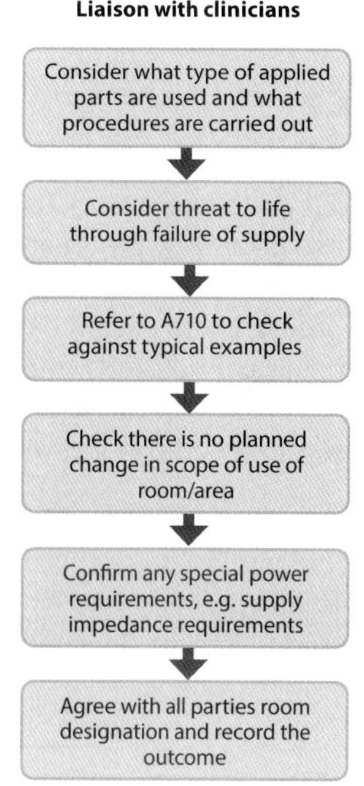

Once determined as a Group 2 medical location it is important to consider the individual factors affecting any design, which include:

(a) requirement to prevent a total loss of supply;
(b) requirements for RCD protection of TN circuits;
(c) additional protection using supplementary equipotential bonding;
(d) reduced touch voltages;
(e) use of medical IT systems;
(f) onerous disconnection times; and
(g) specialist equipment.

20.1 Prevention of loss of supply

Regulation 710.512.1.2 requires that "in the event of a first fault to earth, a total loss of supply in Group 2 shall be prevented."

Initially, this could be interpreted as solely the use of medical IT systems; however, looking further into the international documentation, the note attached to the corresponding regulation refers to this requirement being solved regardless of the medical IT system and management of selectivity, suggesting:

▶ provision of two independent supply lines (see also 710.536.101 of HD 60364-7-710); or
▶ provision of a ring-structure, capable of backing up the mains supply; or
▶ a local additional power supply unit; or
▶ an additional power supply unit for several Group 2 rooms; or
▶ other equally effective technical measures to ensure continuity of mains power.

The requirements could be considered satisfied by applying many of the principles discussed in this Guide and the auto changeover of supplies on loss of supply to an area to allow alternative mains, generator or even UPS backed supplies.

Satisfaction of this requirement is a detailed design decision that will depend on the particular installation, the position of the fault considered and the availability of back up supplies for the designer to include in any final design.

20.2 Use of RCDs

Reading the requirements of BS 7671 to the letter, there are a limited number of instances in Group 2 medical locations where TN circuits are required to have RCD protection. However, by understanding the nuances of Regulation 710.411.4, it is necessary for final circuits in a Group 2 location to be RCD protected unless they are part of an IT system, or unless the equipment intended to be connected to the socket-outlet is not compatible with an RCD, meeting the requirements set out in Regulation 415.1.1. In all instances, the requirements relating to disconnection times and touch voltages between exposed-conductive-parts and extraneous-conductive-parts remains.

As with Group 1 medical locations, RCDs used in Group 2 medical locations must meet the requirements of Regulation 710.411.3.2.5. Type AC RCDs are not permitted due to their inability to detect and ultimately operate effectively, where DC components exist in a waveform.

20.2.1 Operation of RCDs

As with Group 1 medical locations where RCDs are used, it is essential to consider the effects an RCD tripping may have on patient safety. This means ensuring that there are an adequate number of individually protected circuits available in any given area to take account of the total expected equipment leakage currents and the effect a faulty appliance may have on other connected equipment.

20.3 Supplementary equipotential bonding: Group 2 medical locations

▼ **Figure 20.5** Typical theatre configuration

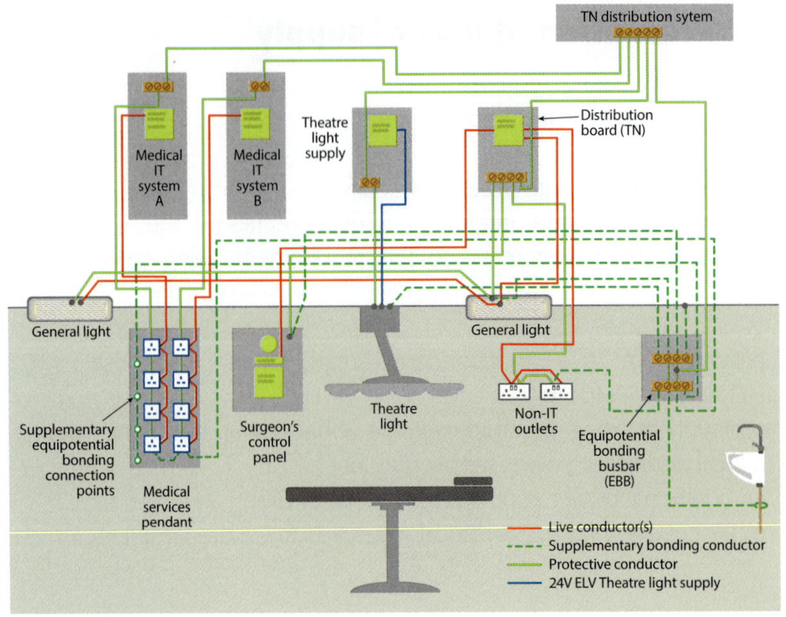

Supplementary equipotential bonding must be applied to the installation in order to meet the requirements of Regulation 710.415.2.1. It is important to note that bonding may not just apply to simultaneously accessible exposed- and extraneous-conductive-parts, but to the items listed in Regulation 710.415.2.1 (note it is the touch voltage requirement that relates to simultaneous accessible parts).

In Group 2 medical locations a maximum value of 0.2 Ω is stated, this is a maximum value which is not to be exceeded. This value should be considered in conjunction with the requirements for a 0.3 s disconnection time (for non RCD protected circuits) as well as the limiting touch voltage of 25 V AC and 60 V DC under fault conditions. Consequently, the important limiting factor is the touch voltage set out in Regulation 710.411.3.2.5, which will affect the size of the protective conductors depending on the rating and type of protective device.

Further detail on supplementary equipotential bonding of Group 2 medical locations and how the size and type of protective device affects the supplementary equipotential bonding is explained in this Guide.

Reduced touch voltage

As with Group 1 locations, Regulation 710.411.3.2.5 sets limiting touch voltage of 25 V AC and 60 V DC under fault conditions using supplementary equipotential bonding.

20.4 Medical IT systems

Medical IT systems are referred to in the industry as isolated power supplies (IPS). Typical examples of locations (usually Group 2 locations) that require the provision of medical IT systems are provided in Annex 710 of BS 7671.

The primary purpose of a medical IT system is to provide a resilient power supply. BS 7671, HTM and SHTM 06-01 all recognise the need for this type of system. These systems are used in medical locations where ME equipment is employed in applications such as intra-cardiac procedures, general surgery or life support intervention where loss of supply would present a danger to life.

The misunderstandings associated with these systems are more than likely linked to the term 'isolated power supply', which gives the impression that the isolation provides electrical protection for the patients and staff. It is understood that the term 'isolated power supply' is commonly used in North America and has been adopted following use in the relevant HTMs and manufacturer data.

The purpose and significant benefit of these systems is to provide first fault resilience, i.e. if an earth fault is created for whatever reason the supply will not be lost. There is a secondary feature of reducing the total earth leakage current to that of the transformer (0.5 mA for this type of transformer).

In terms of electrical supplies to the IT system, it is customary to omit overload protection and provide only short circuit protection between the output of the UPS (if incorporated) and the input to the medical IT system.

▼ **Figure 20.6** Medical IT cabinet (image courtesy of Bender)

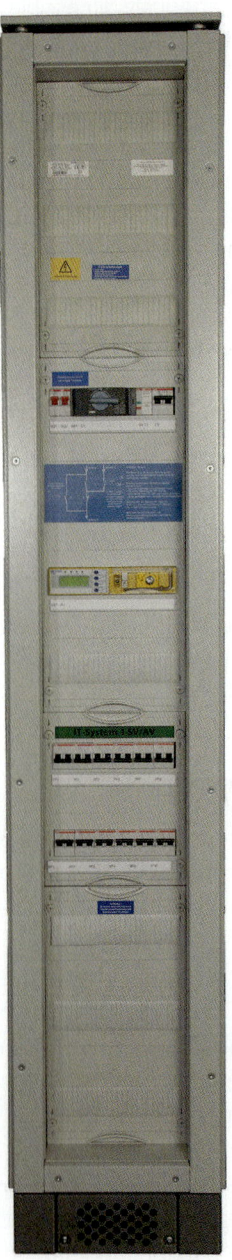

It is usual for systems rated between 4 kVA and 10 kVA (18 A to 44 A) to be protected by Type D circuit-breakers or 63 A or 80 A MCCBs. This prevents the IT system being taken out of service by an overload, which is important as the availability of the supply is paramount to the safety of the patient.

Medical IT systems usually comprise floor-standing distribution cubicles containing 230 V, single phase, 50 Hz isolating transformers (multiple where necessary). These transformers are to comply with BS EN 61558-2-15 with the output isolated from earth.

A medical IT system enclosure is usually positioned in a corridor or cupboard area adjacent to the Group 2 medical location. As the IT system emits heat from the transformer and other components, where the units are contained in cupboards they will require ventilation to prevent excessive heat gains. On larger schemes these units are sometimes located in plant areas above the Group 2 medical location, and often with the UPS equipment, which usually has cooling or adequate ventilation to keep the batteries within the correct environmental conditions.

Although it is not ideal for these units to be located away from the actual area, the equipment is provided to serve a clinical process not the reverse. Manufacturer's recommend having a maximum cable length in the order of 30 m, which may be achieved by locating an IT system in a plantroom above the Group 2 location. Despite this meeting the cable length recommendation, consideration should be given to the accessibility of the unit for maintenance and servicing staff and to the potential impact of moving the unit away from the point of use in terms of resilience and reliability. To maintain the required level of resilience may involve the use of fire resistant/enhanced cabling to compensate for the effects of fire where cables serve equipment in other, adjacent fire compartments etc.

The location of these units in remote areas is not ideal or in the spirit of the manufacturer's recommendations as effectively the medical IT system is ultimately a distribution board and should be readily accessible.

20.5 Alarm annunciator

Upon the detection of a fault condition (overload, over-temperature, earth fault etc.) the staff in the area should be warned by means of an audio-visual device.

These alarm indicator units are normally placed in the locations where the ME equipment is being used to enable the users to take action when an alarm occurs. Alarm units can be placed in more than one location to bring the alarm condition to others attention. It must be stressed that an alarm in a medical IT cupboard or away from the point of use has limited use and therefore should be supplementary alarms with the primary alarm close to the point of use.

Examples of ideal locations are busy but appropriate areas serving Group 2 medical locations, in nursing stations aligned to the Group 2 location and in theatre areas where they are provided in surgeon's control panels (SCPs), sometimes referred to as theatre control panels (TCP).

▼ **Figure 20.7** Alarm annunciators from different manufacturers (images courtesy of Bender, Starkstrom and Brandon Medical)

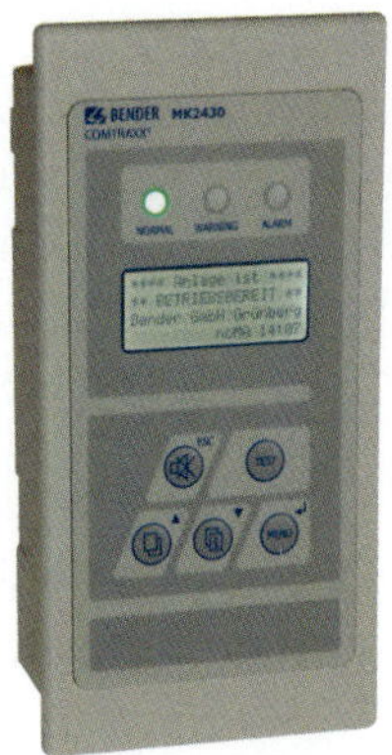
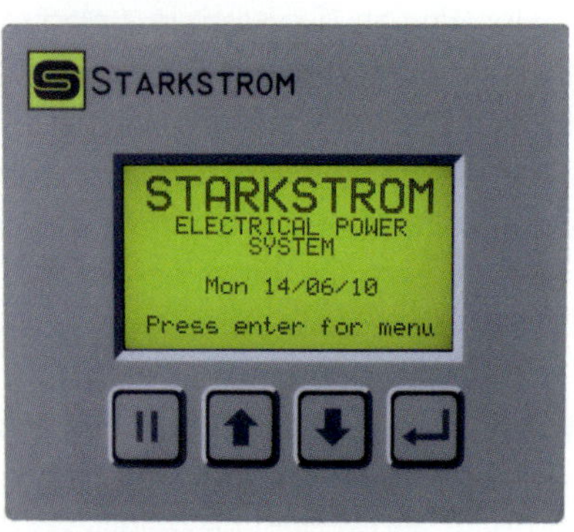

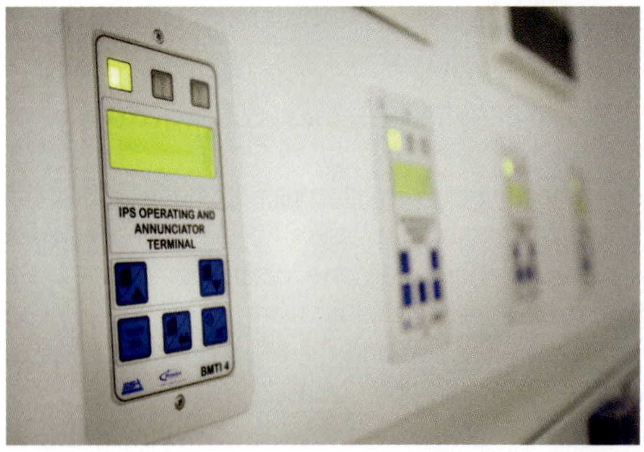

Where alarms are located in surgeon's control panel/theatre control panels (SCP/TCPs), alarms should be such that no master components are located in that SCP/TCP. Where a master unit is necessary, the unit should be a redundant master to allow for complete failure of power to the SCP/TCP without significant effect on the alarm systems.

Each remote alarm panel should incorporate test facilities to allow the system monitor to be interrogated using the self-test function. HTM and manufacturer recommendations suggest that medical IT socket-outlets in rooms should ideally be supplied by multiple transformer arrangements with interleaving of final circuits. As the usual design philosophy is to supply each room from multiple transformer configurations, any remote alarm panel should therefore be capable of clearly reporting alarms for multiple medical IT systems and should have the ability to distinguish faults between systems.

The alarm should be configured to mute the low-level audible alarm by button; however, the indicators on the display will not be able to be reset until the fault has been cleared. If a second fault were to occur during the muted first alarm, the audible alarm should be re-activated. It should be possible to clearly identify each individual fault even if two faults are present concurrently.

In line with the requirements of BS 7671, the annunciator should have a green light to indicate normal operation. In addition, a yellow light and an audible alarm shall indicate 'warning' status should the insulation resistance minimum value be reached or the transformer be overloaded. It should not be possible for the light to be cancelled or disconnected if a fault is present on the system. Finally, a red light shall indicate 'alarm' should the transformer temperature reach a critical value.

20.6 Medical IT system transformers

The IT system transformer must be designed in accordance with BS EN 61558-2-15, providing galvanic isolation between primary and secondary windings.

Galvanic isolation is the principle of **isolating** functional sections of electrical systems to prevent current flow, i.e. no direct conduction path.

These transformers are basic 1:1 transformers, however, they are wound with a slight uplift to bring the voltage back to 230 V on no load. To prevent transformer resonance being amplified by the enclosure the transformer should be mounted on anti-vibration fixings within the system housing.

The transformers have high temperature warnings, however, these warnings should be considered a last defence against failure and as such the transformer may be operating at relatively high temperatures in excess of 100 °C prior to the alarm. Although the transformer is capable of operating in a maximum ambient temperature of 40 °C, the heat emissions from these units can cause heat to rise in unventilated spaces or rooms without cooling. This heat rise will have an effect on all types of equipment including the final circuit MCBs. Details of the effects of temperature are contained in Appendix 7 of this Guide. In addition to the detrimental effects of temperature on the thermal device or other cabling and equipment in the space, the excessive temperatures may appear to the owner operator to be unreasonable or even dangerous. It is therefore desirable to provide cooling or adequate ventilation.

Isolation transformers are monitored for earth leakage by an insulation monitoring device (IMD) that complies with BS EN 61557-8, which, in the event of exceeding specified tolerances, will indicate a fault.

▼ **Figure 20.8** Typical IMD arrangement

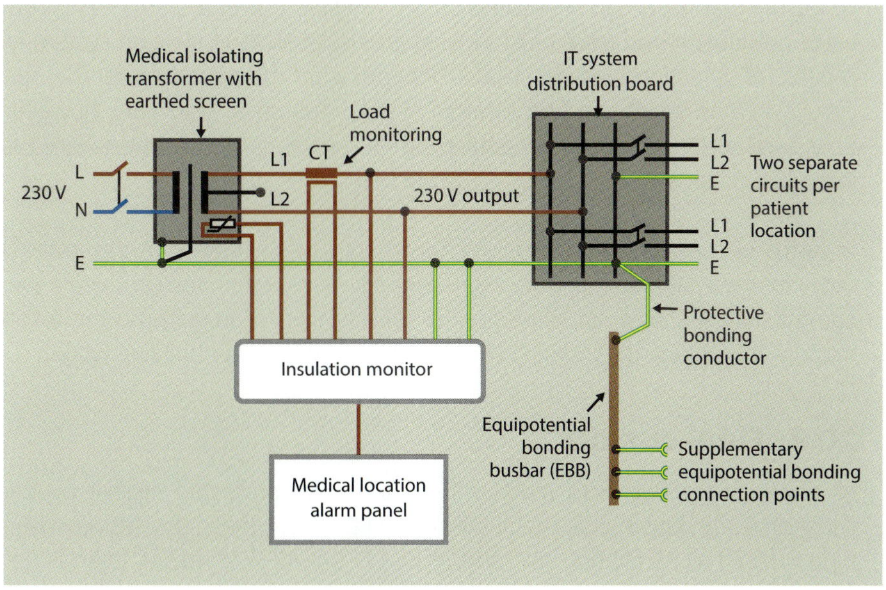

The above IMD is a minimum requirement set out by BS 7671, however, it is recognised that an IT system may serve more than one area and/or the final circuit arrangements may be interleaved with other IT system final circuits to give added resilience.

In such cases as previously indicated, it is usual for the IT systems to cover a wider area than just one room (but should be the same functional group of rooms). It is usual to find that two IT systems serve two adjacent theatres enabling each area to be provided with interleaved final circuits. This arrangement allows a more cost effective solution so that both theatres have a level of resilience with each socket-outlet circuit having an alternative redundant circuit from the alternative medical IT system, rather than providing two separate IT systems for each theatre.

The drawback to this configuration is that a fault on one theatre will be seen as a fault on the IMD, which will cause an alarm in two areas, thus doubling the nuisance to users – for example, personnel in both areas believe they have a fault. Although the alarm occurring in both areas cannot be eradicated as it is a function of the IMD operating, the nuisance effect can be reduced by adding individual circuit insulation fault location system which are also known as earth fault detection systems (EDS).

20.7 Insulation fault location systems (Earth fault detection systems)

In order to enhance the fault identification to the end user it is usual to provide an insulation fault location system, which is often referred to as an earth fault detection system (EDS). This enables individual circuit faults to be identified, thus minimising the nuisance effect to the end user.

An insulation fault location system in accordance with BS EN 61557-9, when fitted, allows faults to be traced and identified automatically, and displayed in text on the associated alarm/display panels that have been specified, without any requirements for circuit isolation and/or manual interrogation by maintenance staff. An example of such a display may be: 'Earth Fault IPS1 Theatre 2 pendant 2 CCT 2.1'.

To ensure that faults can be located on the multiple power systems described above, each individual transformer must include an insulation fault location system, which is capable of detecting individual faults. Depending on the manufacturer the number of circuits that an insulation fault location system can cover may vary, however, these units tend to be provided in modular format, enabling them to be tailored for each individual circuit in use.

In terms of messages, it is usual for designers to be unaware of the exact labelling detail for the systems, so it is therefore useful to have, within the contract in the clinical commissioning stages, an allowance for the installer to programme the text to 'user friendly/appropriate description' following the completion of building works.

20.8 Final circuits

All final-circuit wiring from medical IT systems are protected against overload and short-circuit by double-pole circuit-breakers. Historically, these devices have been 20 A type B MCBs to BS EN 60898-1 and/or BS EN 60947-2. However, there is no reason why a designer should not select a different value of protective device to meet the load requirements and, in particular, Regulation 533.2.1, which requires the correct selection of protective devices to avoid unintentional operation of the protective device due to peak current values being experienced. Further information is contained in Appendices 7 and 8 of this Guide and in IET Guidance Note 5.

As there is no connection to earth for either conductor, they are referred to as L1 and L2, i.e. neither is referred to as the phase or the neutral. However, in accordance with HTM 06-01:2007, these cables are required to be both brown and labelled L1 and L2, with L2 being connected into the neutral of the medical IT socket-outlet. This convention is also referenced in Chapter 9 of IET Guidance Note 7, although this is not expressly stated in BS 7671.

BS 7671 requires that there is no overload protection included in the primary or secondary circuit of the medical IT transformer; instead, it is a requirement that the transformer be monitored for overload and high temperature (see Regulation 710.411.6.3.2). This approach gives the users the opportunity to be 'aware' of overloads or impending problems without necessarily having the outage that is caused when overload protection is operated.

Although the supply to the medical IT system may be set so as to have no overload protection, historically, individual final circuits have been protected by overcurrent protective devices. HTM/SHTM have suggested 20 A type B MCBs, however, the final selection of each final circuit is the choice of the designer, based on load characteristics, as designers have a responsibility to ensure that Regulation 533.2.1 has been satisfied with respect to steady stage and inrush characteristics.

The protective devices connected to the output of the IT transformer give overload and short-circuit protection to the individual final circuit.

Although the common theme of protection around these systems has been the creation of a warning rather than the taking of action, it is necessary on the final circuits to give an amount of protection. In order to minimise the impact of a fault or to give the users/operators warning, the IMD offers that level of warning about first earth faults. In terms of overloads or short circuits, the design is such that all areas have an alternative circuit that supplies additional sockets.

It is common but not mandatory for there to be a redundant circuit, i.e. that there is a 50 % over-provision of socket-outlets in any Group 2 medical location that uses medical IT circuits. This allows for the failure of one circuit.

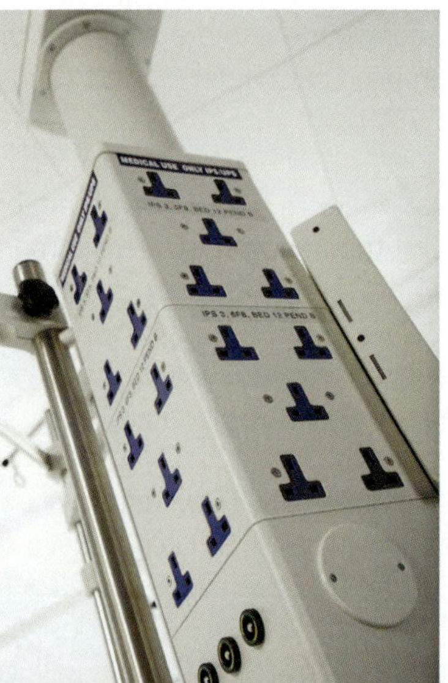

▼ **Figure 20.9** Articulated medical pendant and a different pendant indicating two IT circuits (images courtesy of Bender and Brandon Medical)

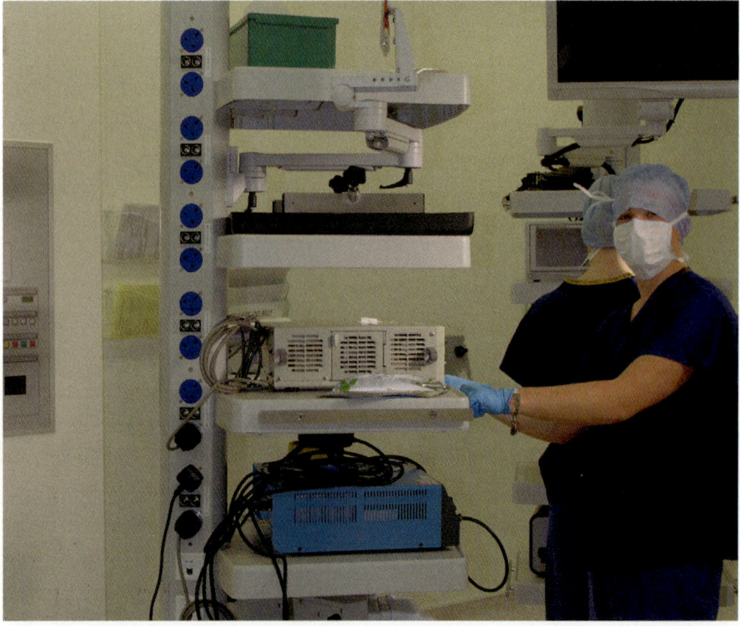

Although this philosophy of redundancy is not clearly detailed in any publications, this philosophy has become commonplace.

In practical terms, to save on a few socket-outlets and final circuit cabling undermines the infrastructure and back-up that is required for a Group 2 location right at the point of delivery.

The provision of additional socket-outlets will need to be balanced against the opportunity for users to accidentally overload a circuit by the way the equipment is 'plugged in' i.e. that one circuit is excessively used rather than the load being distributed more evenly across different final circuits. This is a challenge for both designers and operational managers. The solution to this is normally education, training and clear labelling.

As well as considering the number of socket-outlets, it is important to note that the majority of medical equipment suppliers provide the equipment with shrouded plug tops. These moulded cable restraints can often create challenging scenarios where there are multiple outlets on a particular plate. Those designing and accepting the handover of these systems should ensure that all socket-outlets are usable without one socket-outlet 'fouling' another.

Designers and clients/end users should be aware of this when specifying socket-outlet types and numbers. Those receiving these types of units on behalf of the client should look at availability and usability of the socket-outlets when a number are in use.

▼ **Figure 20.10** Double socket-outlets on rigid pendant arrangement (image courtesy of Starkstrom)

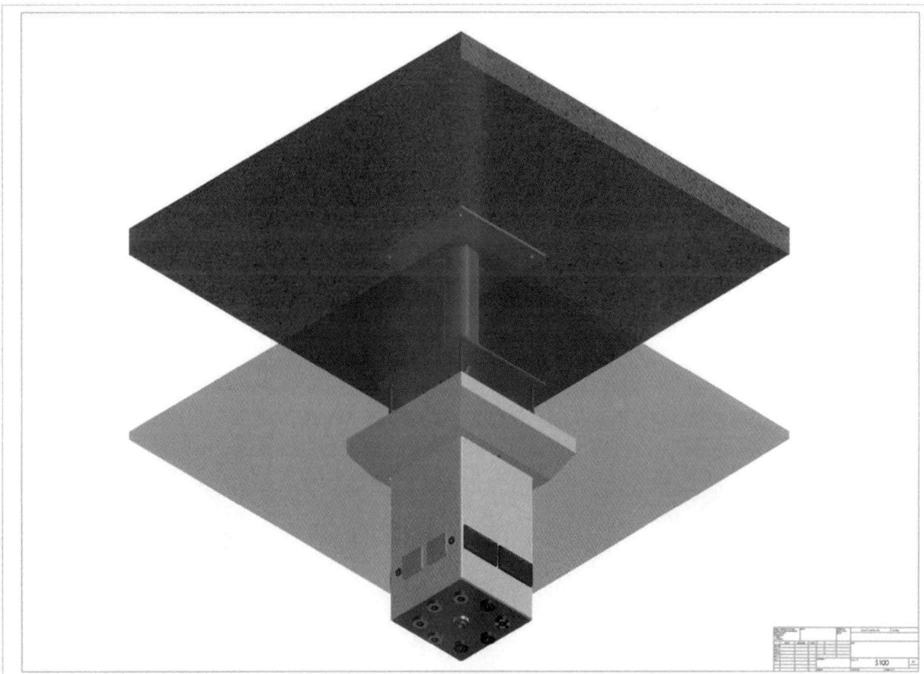

20.9 TN circuits from medical IT cabinets

Often there is a requirement to have a UPS-backed supply (non-medical IT system supply), which does not have to be isolated from earth. This arrangement should ideally be supplied from a dedicated UPS distribution board, which is commonly available where medical IT systems are used.

In other instances, where it is impractical to access a UPS distribution board, another alternative may be a TN circuit fed from the non-IT side of the medical IT system. The added benefit of utilising a small number of low power circuits from the TN side of the IT system is that, where automatic transfer switched are employed, the TN circuit will gain the benefit of the automatic changeover device. The latter option would need to be a bespoke agreement with the manufacturer.

When providing this type of circuit, it is important to remember that this will compound the 'grouping' issues identified earlier relating to circuit-breaker and cable grouping.

These 'local' TN circuits should be restricted in size, serving a small number of points or to serve the SCP/TCP, depending on its configuration. If, however, large picture archiving and communication systems (PACs) viewers and additional screens are envisaged, the UPS circuit should be taken from the main UPS distribution board. The TN circuits are usually available for low-value circuits. Large TN loads should be avoided as they may only serve to destabilise the cable protection that is in place for the medical IT unit supply.

20.10 Medical IT socket-outlets

In order to separate medical IT socket-outlets from other socket-outlets, the current practice is to provide unswitched socket-outlets that are coloured blue with a label or marking stating:

'Medical Equipment Only' in line with Regulation 710.553.1

This format means that the socket-outlet for ME equipment is easily identified from general socket-outlets, which also goes some way into satisfying the requirements of Regulation 710.560.5.7 relating to identification of outlets according to their classification.

▼ **Figure 20.11** Ease of identification on trunking layout (images courtesy of Cableflow International Limited)

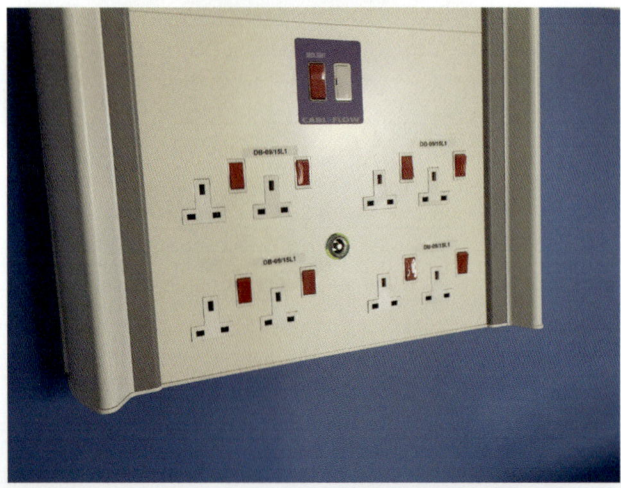

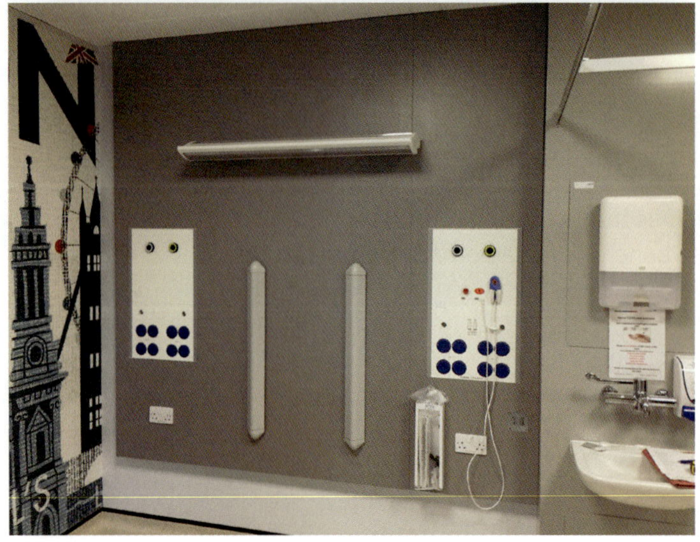

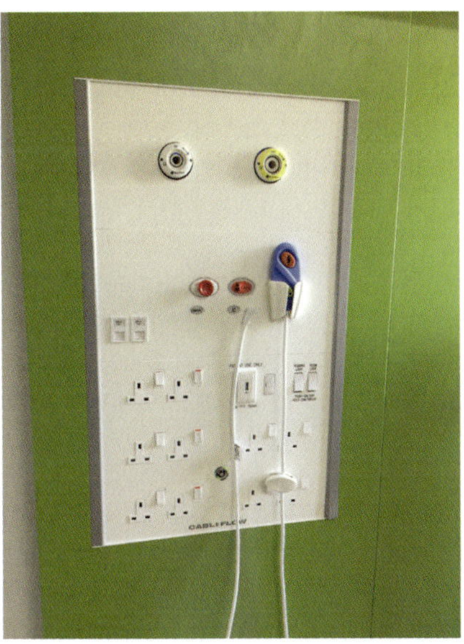

Medical IT final circuits have, in most instances, a higher level of resilience because they are usually configured with a larger number of socket-outlets coupled with interleaving, which gives a level of redundancy beyond those standard TT or TN arrangements.

20.11 Isolated earth pin socket-outlets

The original MEIGaN concept (which is now withdrawn) was to provide isolated earth pin socket-outlets (sometimes referred to as clean earth socket-outlets), in other words, no direct connectivity between the earthed socket-outlet screws on the front plate and the earth pin on the BS 1363 socket-outlet arrangement. This philosophy was to isolate all exposed- and extraneous-conductive-parts from each other. MEIGaN used this approach as a method of reducing stray currents that would usually be picked up through the building structure and the back boxes and were, in turn, earthed separately at what MEIGaN referred to as an ERB (EBB in BS 7671).

BS 7671 and the designers involved with the relevant Working Groups do not advocate the onerous task of carrying out MEIGaN style earthing and bonding on the basis that it is onerous and, in the majority of cases, unnecessary. It is also costly, confusing and, in many cases, the cause of unwanted stress amongst installers and verifiers.

Any benefit of the isolated earth pin arrangement is potentially nullified through fortuitous connections with extraneous-conductive-parts that have common connections, such as metallic brackets and framework, to the services as they enter the location. However, in a correctly installed BS 7671-complaint installation, the effects of isolated earth pin systems are hardly noticeable, leaving the benefits of such a system highly questionable.

Finally, if the designer has to change the characteristics of the protective device, it will be necessary to have very low impedances (which may not be achievable) in order to meet the touch voltage limitations in Regulation 710.411.3.2.5. Consequently, this approach to isolated earth configuration may not be sustainable.

20.12 Number of socket-outlets per final circuit

There are various figures recommended by suppliers of medical IT systems as to the number of socket-outlets that can be applied to a final circuit. In reality, it is for designers to consider the potential loading and the likelihood that an individual circuit could be overloaded.

This is also important where circuits are interleaved, as it may be possible that staff have particular preferences for positions, leaving all 'A' supplies loaded with 'B' supplies unused, when the designer has intended that both supplies will be used equally. Consideration should therefore be given for circuit references and layout at design stage.

A requirement of Regulation 710.531.2.4 is to ensure that the circuit is not subject to excessive earth leakage currents that may flow on the protective conductor under normal conditions. This should be designed to be minimal on all circuits, including medical IT systems and on TN installations.

When providing socket-outlets for any type of circuit it is important that there is sufficient flexibility in the number and position of the socket-outlets to ensure that individual circuits are not overloaded.

It is also important that there are no compatibility elements with the load and the circuit protective conductor, for example, harmonics, inrush current etc.

20.12.1 Do I need two medical IT systems for every Group 2 location?

The simple answer is no. If, for example, you have a single Group 2 location, such as an interventional X-ray room, a single medical IT supply is sufficient as long as it can cope with the expected load. However, it is important to provide two individual final circuits feeding several socket-outlets as Regulation 710.553.1(ii) states. This is often misinterpreted as the requirement for multiple medical IT systems.

20.13 What is the maximum length of run of an IT circuit?

There has been much confusion about the length of run of a final circuit to a number of medical IT socket-outlets. Followers of MEIGaN will be familiar with the restrictive length of run for protective conductors or protective bonding conductors. The limiting factor of 0.1 Ω described in MEIGaN meant that, in simple terms, 6 mm^2 protective or bonding conductors could not be longer than 31 m or shorter for a 4 mm^2 equivalent conductor. This figure was then confused with the maximum length of run of an IT circuit.

The majority of cables will be 4 mm^2 radial circuits as the 20 A ring circuit is not a standard circuit configuration. The limiting factor may be due to load and the ability of the protective device to operate without exceeding temperature or energy let-through requirements.

In a standard circuit design there are obvious limitations on the length of runs, and these will determine values such as volt drop, disconnection times etc. These values can be corroborated through simple calculation, usually using proprietary software, which usually focuses on maximum Z_s values to meet disconnection times. However, as proprietary software does not directly deal with IT systems, an alternative approach needs to be taken.

Looking at the challenges for a designer, they are faced with the fact that a medical IT system is so designed that it does not fail on first fault to earth, so the usual concept of disconnection times for TN systems is not applicable.

Chapter 41 of BS 7671 deals with this by requiring IT systems that do not disconnect the supply on first fault by having warning measures, which is augmented in Section 710.

Where a supply does not disconnect upon first fault, it effectively means that the system has now temporarily become a TN system. Regulation 411.6.4 requires that an IT system where the midpoint conductor is not distributed (as it is with a medical IT system) is able to meet the following requirements:

$$Z_s \leq \frac{U \times C_{min}}{2I_a}$$

where:

U   is the nominal AC rms or DC voltage, in volts, between line conductors.

Z_s is the impedance in ohms of the fault loop, comprising the line conductor and the protective conductor of the circuit.

I_a is the current in amps (A) causing operation of the protective device within the time specified in Table 41.1 of Regulation 411.3.2.2, or as appropriate, Regulation 411.3.2.3, for a TN system.

C_{min} is the minimum voltage factor to take account of voltage variations depending on time and place, changing of transformer taps and other considerations. The value used is currently 0.95.

▼ **Figure 20.12** Medical IT system fault

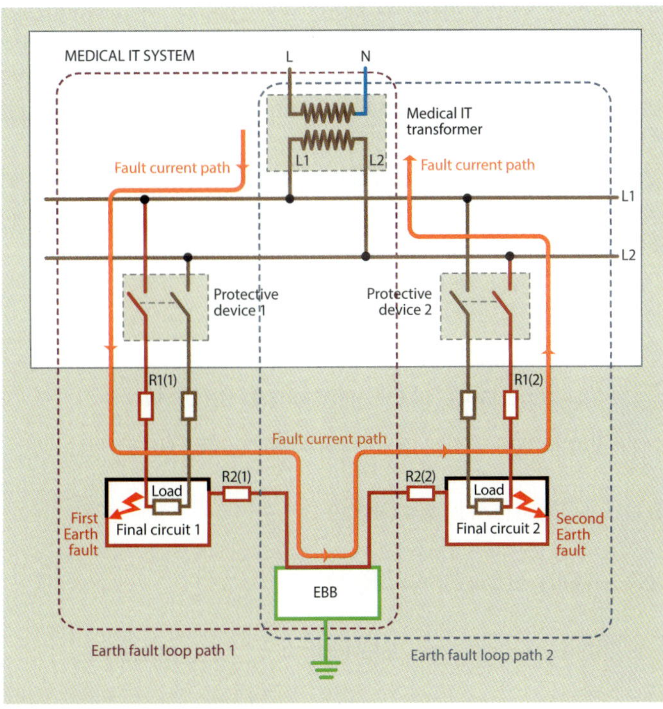

Figure 20.12 indicates the potential earth fault loop created as earth faults occur on medical IT systems. This has always caused an element of confusion as, technically, with an isolated system there is no Z_s. However, in a healthy circuit, considering the following scenario, the term Z_s is applicable even if it's not in the usual context.

The resulting fault current is as indicated in Figure 20.13.

▼ **Figure 20.13** Resulting fault current

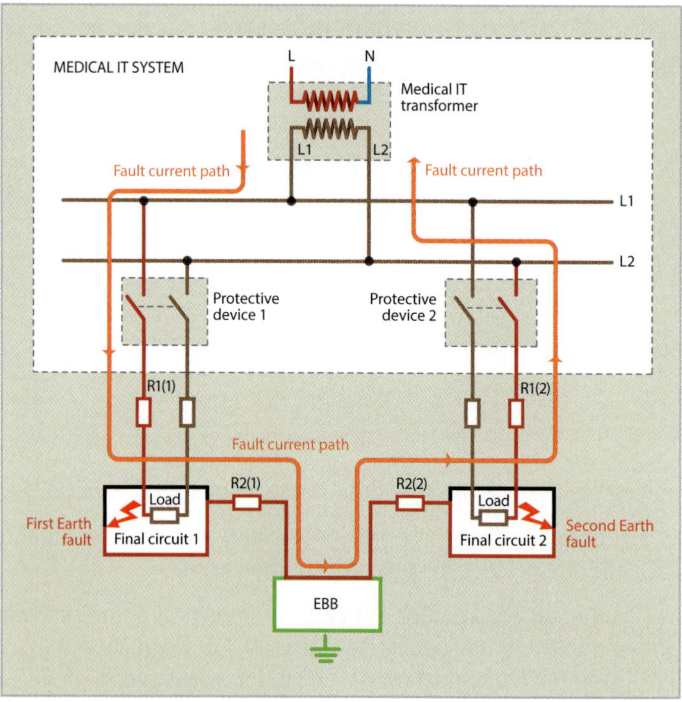

We can therefore see that there is an earth fault loop that is comprised of the impedance of:

(a) the secondary winding (which effectively would be Z_e);
(b) L1 to the point of fault (which would be R1(1) in the diagram);
(c) L2 to the point of fault (which would be R1(2)in the diagram); and
(d) the earth path in the diagram, which would be between the points of fault and, in a Group 2 medical location, would be through the protective conductors and the supplementary equipotential bonding conductor for that location.

Relating the values back to the standard formula as above, we would find that:

$$Z_s = Z_e + (R1+R2)$$

where:

Z_e is the impedance of the transformer secondary.

LOR   is the length of run of the cable in metres (m).

$$R1 = (R1(1) \times LOR) + (R1(2) \times LOR) \ \Omega$$

$$R2 = (R2(1) \times LOR) + (R2(2) \times LOR) \ \Omega$$

We can use the manufacturer's data to find Z_s, for example:

Z of 10 kVA transformer = 0.158 Ω

Z of 8 kVA transformer = 0.198 Ω

I_a for a 20 A Type B MCB = 100 A

I_a for a 20 A Type C MCB = 200 A

Consequently, applying the formula in Regulation 411.6.4 for a 20 A type B device with a 10 kVA transformer gives the following maximum Z_s:

$$Z_s = \frac{230 \times 0.95}{2 \times 100A} = \textbf{1.0925}$$

Using the same transformer with a 20 A Type C MCB:

$$Z_s = \frac{230 \times 0.95}{2 \times 200A} = \textbf{0.54625} \; \Omega$$

Using the same transformer with a 20 A Type D MCB:

$$Z_s = \frac{230 \times 0.95}{2 \times 400A} = \textbf{0.2731} \; \Omega$$

Using the 20 A type B results:

$$Z_s = 1.0925 = Z_e + (R1+R2)$$

Resulting in (R1+R2) = 1.0925-0.158= **0.9345** Ω

If the maximum impedance for any exposed-conductive-part or extraneous-conductive-part to the equipotential bonding busbar (EBB) is for the purpose of these calculations 0.1 Ω (set out by previous guidance and does not necessarily provide compliance with Regulation 710.411.3.2.5 for all protective device types) then the R2 maximum value would be 0.2 Ω.

Applying this to the formula:

R1 = 0.9345-0.2 = **0.7345** Ω

As the formula in Regulation 411.6.4 uses the factor $2 \times I_a$ it takes into account that there are two circuits involved. The R1 impedance divided by the length of run (LOR) will therefore provide the theoretical maximum cable length (subject to volt drop, energy let-through and capacitive coupling limitations).

Using the 70 °C copper cable values from IET Guidance Note 1 we can see the following values for Ohms per metre of cable at a particular size:

2.5 mm = 0.0889 Ω/m, 4 mm= 0.0553 Ω/m, 6 mm = 0.037 Ω/m

Consequently, if R1 consists of a 4.0 mm² cable, this would give a maximum theoretical length of:

Max LOR = 0.7345/0.00553 = **132.8 m**

(Subject to capacitive coupling, volt drop and energy let-through limitations of the device in conjunction with the current withstand capacity of the cables and equipment.)

If we use the same equipment but using the 20 A type C devices we find the following:

$$Z_s = \frac{230 \times 0.95}{2 \times 200A} = \textbf{0.54625} \; \Omega$$

Applying the above formula we find that the value for R1 is now **0.34625** Ω

This equates to a theoretical **62 m** maximum length of run using 4.0 mm² cable.

If a smaller value of transformer is used the corresponding increase in impedance of the transformer will affect the LOR available for the designer to use.

Having obtained a theoretical LOR we still need to satisfy touch voltage requirements of Regulation 710.411.3.2.5, which limits the touch voltage on simultaneously accessible parts to 25 V. This process is detailed in the additional supplementary equipotential bonding section of this Guide.

As can be seen, the limiting value suggested in HTM 06-01:2007 is not due to the volt drop on the protective conductors. It relates to accessibility, the potential to create excessive capacitive coupling of the cables forming the overall system and, ultimately, the fault loop created when two separate (different) conductors on the IT system become connected to earth under fault conditions. The final detail is for the designer to consider/work out, taking into account circuit and environmental conditions.

In summary, this Guide does not advocate that designers should extend all the medical IT system circuits to maximum permissible lengths, as there may be other factors that affect the design and, ultimately, compliance. It also does not suggest that medical IT system cabinets 'have' to be located in the medical location, which may compromise clinical functionality.

As with most design scenarios, the design of medical locations is often a balance of a number of factors. What this Guide intends to demonstrate is that there is no definite one size fits all solution. It is the responsibility of the designer to consider all the relevant factors in each individual installation design.

20.14 Can I only use 20 A type B MCBs on medical IT systems?

The design of any installation is the responsibility of the designer. In Group 2 locations, the selection of protective device is believed by many designers to be fixed, i.e. as indicated in HTM 06-01:2007 (SHTM for Scotland). This approach is contrary to any requirements of BS 7671 and the aim of this Guide.

It is the responsibility of the designer to select the appropriate protective device for a particular installation. In the design of socket-outlet circuits, their exact use is often unknown. The design of socket-outlet circuits normally involves the designer receiving information about equipment and use from the client and then making a decision relating to loading, starting currents harmonics and other system and waveform pollutants. Regulation 533.2.1 requires designers to choose current settings in accordance with Regulation 433.1 and also to consider prevention of unintentional operation of the protective device due to peak current values.

The protective device should be selected so that it is suitable for the design load and the equipment that would be reasonably expected to be used on that final circuit.

Often the designer is driven to use a 20 A type B BS EN 60898-1 device through the belief that the HTM or SHTM has directed them to do so. This belief can be incorrect: HTMs provide guidance only. Although HTM or SHTM compliance may be mandated in a contract, the parties are often able to, firstly, deviate from HTMs in the contract stage to seek cost savings. Secondly, and more importantly, make appropriate choices including escalation to the client where necessary if there is an incompatibility between the guidance and the equipment as supplied from the client.

There is an added misconception throughout the industry that manufacturers will only provide IT circuits with type B circuit-breakers. Medical IT system suppliers will usually supply the standard protective devices. However, it is the duty of the designer to specify to the manufacturer the correct protective device characteristics.

In reality, manufacturers will supply what is required as part of the design and will have, on occasion, supplied Type C and Type D circuit-breakers to overcome the unwanted tripping of MCBs where inrush current is significant.

20.15 Do we need to provide TN socket-outlets in a Group 2 medical location?

The straightforward answer is yes.

In a Group 2 medical location there is a requirement to provide socket-outlets supplied from a medical IT system. The question that is often asked is: why do we not supply all socket-outlets in a Group 2 location from a medical IT system? The simple answer is cost and compatibility.

If all socket-outlets were supplied from the IT system, the cost would increase significantly when modifying or adding socket-outlets to power final circuits. This increase is not restricted to additional cabling but will have a significant impact on equipment and infrastructure.

The increase in infrastructure would potentially include medical IT units, alarms and UPS back-ups etc. causing unnecessary construction costs. In addition to the electrical equipment cost burden, there would be an architectural impact in terms of space and the structural limitations on floors to support heavy battery racks.

These added requirements would be necessary for lots of equipment that do not require that level of resilience and are not necessarily compatible with that equipment.

Compatibility in terms of the many items of equipment, including imaging equipment, would have excessive current demands, causing a temporary overload scenario in the medical IT system. Additionally, they may operate circuit-breakers that are provided for overcurrent protection due to overloading or simply inrush current from specific equipment. This, and the unnecessary physical burden placed on the layout in terms of UPS and IT cabinets, makes the matter impractical.

Almost all Group 2 medical locations may require the services of a mobile X-ray unit, either to take static images or to provide dynamic moving images (fluoroscopy). The power requirements for these units, although connected to a standard 13 A socket-outlet, can easily overload the medical IT system, especially systems that require a short 10 mS to 300 mS high current, low impedance source.

A mobile fluoroscopy X-ray unit may require greater than 2 kW for extended periods of time (from a couple of seconds to 30 minutes), which will easily overload most medical IT transformers and endanger the other life-critical equipment.

Given that a mobile X-ray unit is not often considered critical to life safety, it may be prudent to consider the provision of a dedicated mains socket-outlet for the connection of mobile X-ray equipment to Group 2 medical locations. Further consideration should be made about the availability of this equipment in terms of whether a no-break supply is required. If deemed necessary, this may be made available through either a dedicated or central UPS to suit the design conditions.

Consideration should also be given to the connection of non-medical electrical equipment that may be required for use in Group 2 medical locations, such as cleaning equipment.

Where such a TN supply socket-outlet is made available in Group 2 medical locations it must be RCD protected and its purpose must be clearly marked. An example of suitable marking is given in Figure 20.14 (note how the yellow background adds to the prominence).

▼ **Figure 20.14** Example marking for TN-S socket used in Group 2 medical locations

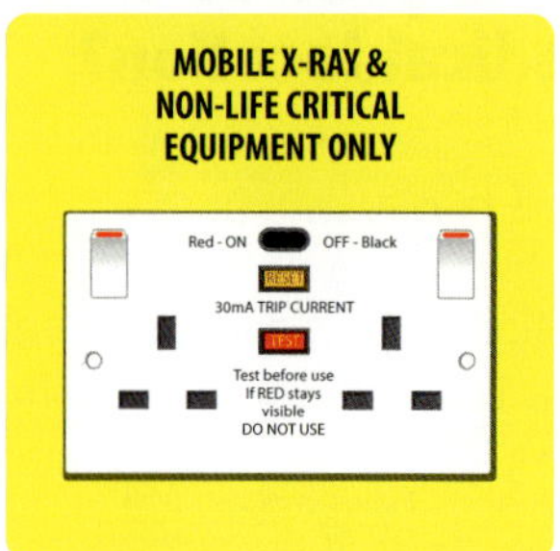

Even a Group 2 location that consists of a permanently installed X-ray system should consider having such a socket-outlet to allow for the use of a back-up, mobile X-ray system to be available for use in the event of a breakdown of the primary equipment.

20.16 Surgeon's control panels (SCPs)

The surgeon's control panel is typically based on a standard design but the final control, alarms and indicators, and associated programming of PLCs are usually bespoke to the particular project. This device allows the surgeon to have information about all sorts of alarms and interfaces that they may not wish to control but probably need to be aware of. This panel is also known as a theatre control panel (TCP) by some in the industry and the two terms appear to be interchangeable.

Surgeon's control units come in a variety of formats. Today, the 'traditional' surgeon's control panel, which was typically made from stainless steel, with knobs, dials and indicator lights, has been replaced with membrane-type panels or even electronic software-driven touch-sensitive screens, very much along the tablet format that is currently dominating the markets.

▼ **Figure 20.15** Rear access traditional SCP (image courtesy of Brandon Medical)

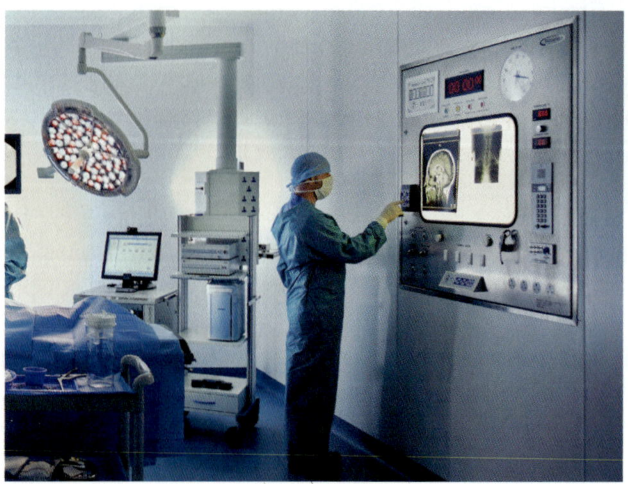

Unlike medical devices that need to conform to the Medical Device Directive or BS EN 60601, the SCP is a bespoke piece of equipment differing from project to project. If this is treated as a medical device, there would need to be a large amount of testing and assurances that are generally unnecessary and would require an equivalent process of type testing. As such, if the client specified a panel and functionality and thereafter was to change its function, the panel would need a new assessment. This approach is obviously cost restrictive and hence there has been no drive to bring SCPs into the scope of any particular standard.

> **Note:** Where an SCP provides socket-outlets then the requirements of the Medical Supply Units to BS EN 11197 may be applicable.

If the client specified a panel and functionality and thereafter was to change its function, the panel would need a new assessment. This approach is obviously cost restrictive and hence there has been no drive to bring SCPs into the scope of any particular standard, although at the time of writing, a standard for SCPs was under consideration.

However, when specifying and accepting a surgeon's panel, which is in or adjacent to the patient environment, it is important to ensure that the signal colour coding meets the requirements of BS EN 60601.

Red	Warning – immediate response by the OPERATOR is required
Yellow	Caution – prompt response by the OPERATOR is required
Green	Ready for use
Any other colour	Meaning is other than that for red, yellow or green

The term 'any other colour' relates to the fact that red, yellow and green are reserved for the functions identified above.

There are a number of options available to ensure that these units are electrically powered in accordance with the requirements of Section 710, including powering from:

(a) a PELV supply with an RMS Voltage of 25 V AC or 60 V DC or less;
(b) an IT system with appropriate monitoring (not necessarily the IT supplies); and
(c) a TN supply with an RCD that complies with Regulation 415.1.1 of BS 7671.

The supply for an SCP is therefore likely to be a 230 V TN supply fed via an RCD. In order to improve the resilience of, and prevent interruptions to, the supply, it is usual to provide the supply on a UPS. This can be done by taking a supply from a UPS distribution board or, if available, fitting an RCBO to the non-isolated section of a medical IT system cabinet.

Where the panel is supplying other services, such as medical gases, it would also need to meet the requirements of BS EN ISO 11197.

20.16.1 Total power failure to the SCP/TCP

In determining the level of resilience required for a particular piece of equipment or system, asking a simple question such as 'what happens if...?' normally will reveal a number of answers which will provide the enquirer with a route to achieving compliance.

Asking this type of question may seem pessimistic, however, it is particularly useful when planning any resilient system or looking to avoid the pitfalls of being caught out not knowing what is happening or what has to happen to resolve a situation. I am often surprised to find that no one else has asked that question. Therefore, when I am involved in resilience planning, I always encourage everyone to challenge, as experience has shown that simple omissions or oversight can have devastating consequences.

As part of the research for this Guide, I asked suppliers throughout the industry 'what happens if...?' on most products and components. When the question was applied to SCPs, astonishingly, the answer was not particularly forthcoming, mainly due to the fact that there is very little opportunity for an SCP supply to fail and nobody had perhaps examined the matter rigorously. Following considerable probing of most of the suppliers and assemblers of this equipment the general answer 'not a lot' came back.

Industry belief is that very little will occur except the loss of local control and loss of alarm interfaces as most of the equipment controlled at the SCP can be controlled by its local control, so loss of supply in most scenarios is not catastrophic.

In order to avoid potential catastrophic breakdown, a number of simple actions can be taken when specifying SCPs:

(a) ensure that the SCP powers as little of the external equipment as is practical;

(b) specify equipment and interfaces so that there is a fall-back/emergency control that is not located in the SCP; and

(c) specify that any 'master units' shall not be solely used in the SCP and, where the master unit functionality is required by that service, ensure that a redundant master arrangement is specified. This will then prevent major system failure and retain a level of functionality elsewhere if the need arises.

Although the SCP is a useful central point for theatre activities, it should be designed, installed and commissioned to be as resilient as possible. Consequently, where that simple problem of component failure may cause an RCD to operate, by taking the time to ask and understand how the panel will operate the equipment that is connected to it will go a long way to ensuring that there are no crises and that a fall-back solution is readily available.

This is done through close liaison with suppliers and the users of equipment so that, if the worst should happen, all parties know what to do to mitigate the consequences and, importantly, how to rectify the fault and bring back normal operation.

It should be noted, that at the time of publication, a Code of Practice for SCP/TCPs was in an early stage of drafting by the Specialist Ventilation Group of CIBSE.

Inspection and testing   21

21.1 General requirements

Regulation 134.2.1 states: "During erection and on completion of an installation or an addition or alteration to an installation, and before it is put into service, appropriate inspection and testing shall be carried out by competent persons to verify that the requirements of this Standard have been met."

This regulation requires that all installations should be inspected by persons competent in inspection and testing, i.e., a person who has sufficient training, experience and knowledge to carry out the testing effectively and safely.

This would normally involve the person having a recognised qualification, such as City & Guilds 2394/5, or historically 2391, along with sufficient experience in medical locations installations to carry out effective inspection and testing. This does not necessarily mean that a specialist testing course or training module is required to be competent in testing and inspecting medical locations.

Although the responsibility for the comparison of inspection and test results, with respect to the relevant criteria, lies with the installing/inspection and testing organisation, there is a requirement on other stakeholders, including the designers and manufacturer/suppliers, to provide the relevant information to allow certification in line with BS 7671.

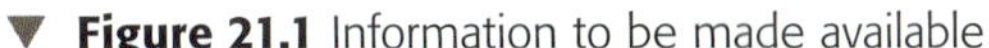

▼ **Figure 21.1** Information to be made available

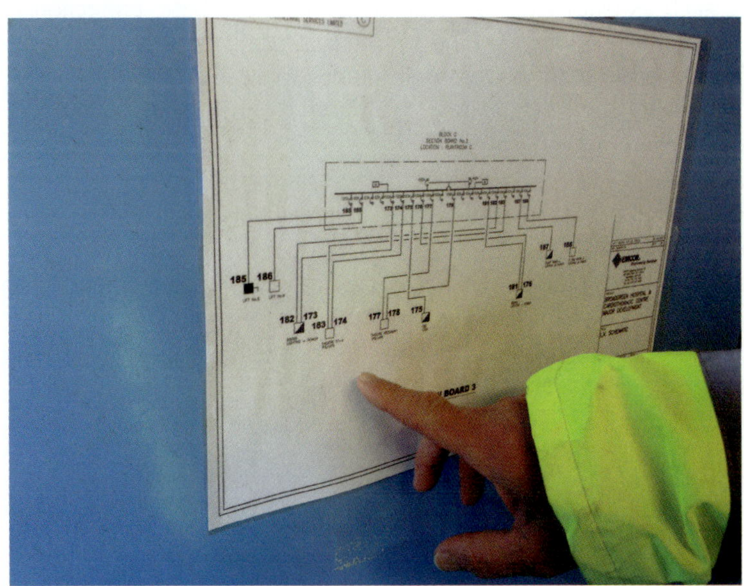

© The Institution of Engineering and Technology

This information should be available for all sources of supply and include:

(a) diagrams, charts or tables;

(b) the maximum demand, expressed in amperes, kW or kVA per phase (after diversity is taken into account);

(c) the number and type of live conductors of the source(s) of energy and of the circuits used in the installation;

(d) the type of earthing arrangement(s) used by the installation;

(e) the nominal voltage(s) and characteristics, including harmonic distortion;

(f) the nature of the current and supply frequency;

(g) the prospective short-circuit current at the origin of the installation;

(h) the earth fault loop impedance (Z_e) of that part of the system external to the installation as appropriate to the location; and

(i) the type and rating of the overcurrent protective device acting at the origin of the installation.

21.2 Initial inspection and testing of medical locations

Initial inspection and testing of medical locations is primarily no different from those of other locations, in that dates and results of verifications in all installations are required to be recorded. This ensures compliance with the EAWR.

Regulation 4(2) of the EAWR 1989 indicates that, by keeping records, including the initial inspection values, the condition of equipment and the effectiveness of maintenance can be monitored.

The *Memorandum of Guidance on the Electricity at Work Regulations 1989* (HSR25) recommends that records of all maintenance, including test results, be kept throughout the life of an installation. This places a duty on the installer and maintainer to provide adequate certification for all new and amended equipment and the owner/occupying authority to maintain and retain adequate records.

The requirements of Chapter 61 must be followed, with obvious exceptions of those items, such as placing out of reach, which provides basic protection against electric shock and which are not permitted in medical locations. In fact, the test regime should verify that these prohibited methods are not applicable:

(a) connection of conductors;

(b) identification of conductors;

(c) routing of cables in safe zones, or protection against mechanical damage, in compliance with Section 522;

(d) selection of conductors for current-carrying capacity and voltage drop, in accordance with the design;

(e) connection of single-pole devices for protection or switching inline conductors only;

(f) correct connection of accessories and equipment;

(g) presence of fire barriers, suitable seals and protection against thermal effects; and

(h) methods of protection against electric shock:

   (i) both basic protection and fault protection, i.e.:
- SELV;
- PELV;
- double insulation; and
- reinforced insulation.

   (ii) basic protection (including measurement of distances, where appropriate)
- i.e. protection by insulation of live parts;
- protection by a barrier or an enclosure;
- protection by obstacles (not permitted in medical locations); and
- protection by placing out of reach (not permitted in medical locations).

The remaining requirements relate to ensuring that the supplementary equipotential bonding conductors are installed in accordance with Regulation 710.415.2.2 of BS 7671 and the values set out by the designer in order to meet Regulation 710.411.3.2.5.

▼ **Figure 21.2** Measurement of values

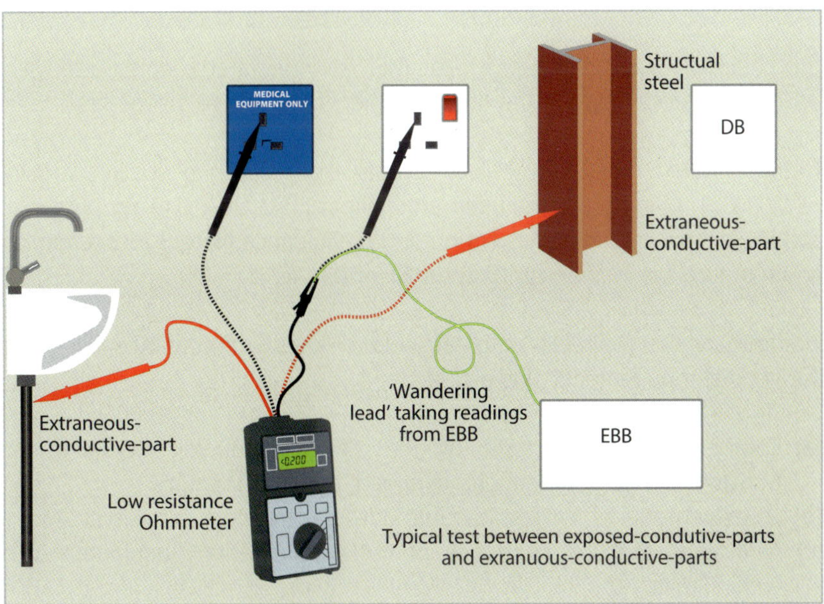

This regulation requires the values to be recorded. This goes above and beyond the normal testing regime requirements of ensuring continuity of the bonding and protective conductors. However, there is limited space to record this information on standard forms.

The checklist below could provide a useful tool when ensuring that compliance and future periodic requirements are met.

▼ **Figure 21.3** Record of resistances

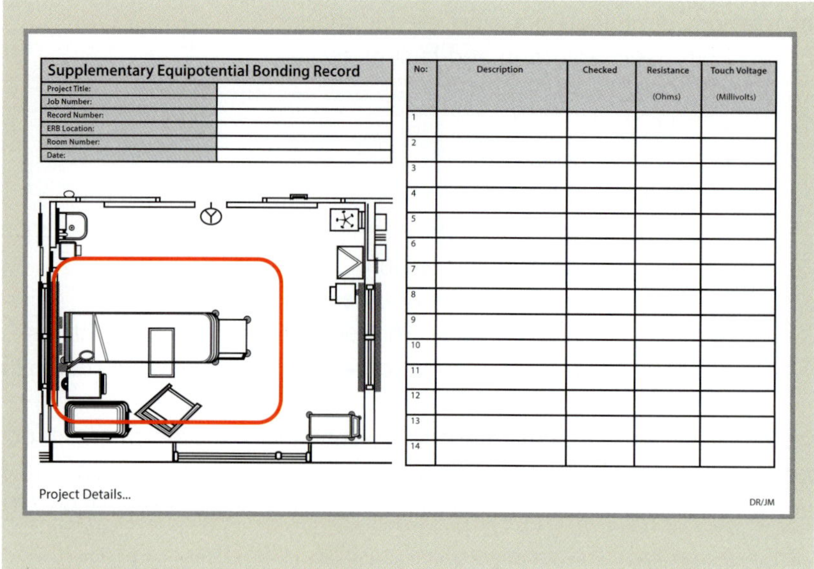

Note: *Thanks to Messers Rowe and McMullen for the reproduction of this form*

This checklist, or a variation of it (less MEIGaN orientated), would also make a useful 'as installed' document for the designer, clients and future inspectors.

There is within Regulation 710.61 a note that relates to specific requirements in HTM 06-01. Many of the requirements within HTM 06-01 relate primarily to testing and inspection procedures as set out in IET Guidance Note 3 *Inspection and Testing*, which in turn are in line with Chapter 61 of BS 7671.

In summary, the contractor is to carry out all tests in accordance with Chapter 61 of the general requirements plus provide:

(a) complete functional tests of the (IMDs) including insulation failure and transformer high temperature, overload, and discontinuity;
(b) measurements of leakage currents of IT transformers in no-load; and
(c) verification that the resistance of the supplementary equipotential bonding is within limits.

In terms of the items above, items (a) and (b) relate to Group 2 locations and should be provided by the medical IT system suppliers as part of their commissioning documentation. However, item (c) can and should be tested by those installing the fixed wiring systems and recorded with the fixed installation wiring documentation.

What is apparent is the lack of suitable 'linking' documentation in terms of model forms to link the healthcare engineering aspects to the standard forms. This is despite the HTM provision of additional test sheets for healthcare engineers or those working on behalf of the healthcare organisation to review certain areas of inspection, including HV equipment that is outside the scope of BS 7671.

It is, therefore, the responsibility of the installing contractor to provide sufficient documentation to link the requirements of a standard electrical installation certificate (EIC) to the additional requirements laid out in BS 7671 for initial certification purposes.

It is also the responsibility of the person receiving the information on behalf of the client/organisation to ensure that there is suitable documentation and 'signposting' within the operation and maintenance information supplied to allow future periodic inspection to take place.

A preliminary check list has been provided in Appendix 9 to assist hand over of Group 2 locations.

21.3 Periodic inspection and testing

Regulation 710.62, unusually, contains no regulatory information, only notes. The general requirement to carry out periodic inspection and testing is contained in Chapter 62 of the main requirements. There are specific notes relating to medical locations, however, the majority of this information relates to the testing of the medical IT systems. The testing of such systems should be carried out by the manufacturer, or those with specific knowledge of testing the insulation monitoring devices (IMDs), the transformer temperatures, overload, discontinuity and the associated alarms.

In terms of the medical IT socket-outlets, these could be tested by the electrical contractor. However, the contractor must take into account the fact that in an IT system, as far as standard electrical equipment is concerned, there is no reference to earth for the mains supply, making the rendering of certain standard tests invalid.

The note also requires an annual inspection of the supplementary equipotential bonding in the particular location to ensure that the values of resistance are within the requirements of Regulation 710.415.2.2 and those set by the designer, which will ensure compliance with Regulation 710.411.3.2.5. Regardless of whether the values are within the prescribed limits, it is important to understand any significant changes. For example, a previous value of 0.06 Ω suddenly increasing to 0.15 Ω would suggest that there is degradation in the connection, which will eventually degrade beyond limits and should be investigated regardless of being within the limits set by the designer.

In summary, for periodic inspection and testing, in addition to the requirements of the general requirements of Chapter 62 the following actions are required:

(a) annually: complete functional tests of the insulation monitoring devices (IMDs).
(b) annually: verify that the resistance of the supplementary equipotential bonding is within limits.
(c) every 3 years: measure leakage current of the output circuit and of the enclosure of the medical IT transformers.

These requirements are supported in IET Guidance Note 3. Extracts are included as follows.

▼ **Table 21.1** Extract of Guidance Note 3 Table 3.2

Hospitals and medical clinics	Routine check	Maximum period between inspections	Notes
Hospitals and medical clinics - general areas	1 year	5 years	1, 2
Hospitals and medical clinics - medical locations	6 months	1 year	9

Notes:

1. Particular attention must be taken to comply with SI 2002 No. 2665 – Electricity Safety, Quality and Continuity Regulations 2002 (as amended).

2. Electricity at Work Regulations 1989, Regulation 4 and Memorandum of guidance (HSR25) published by the HSE.

9. Medical locations shall have their isolating transformer equipment inspected and tested for functionality as well as alarms etc.; every third year the output leakage current of the IT isolating equipment shall be measured.

The healthcare related elements of periodic inspection and testing indicated above are often misinterpreted by organisations. In order to clarify the requirements a revised table is provided in Appendix 11 of this Guide.

21.3.1 Additional documentation

As with the initial verification documentation there is the lack of suitable 'linking' documentation in terms of model forms to link the healthcare engineering aspects to the standard forms.

It is the responsibility of the testing organisation to provide sufficient documentation to link the requirements of an electrical installation condition report (EICR) to the additional recommendations laid out in and supported in IET Guidance Note 3.

The following form is a development of a document initiated by Group Management Ltd. The document is a conceptual document to encourage organisations to develop documentation which meets the relevant requirements and is appropriate to their own organisational needs.

▼ **Figure 21.4** Linking documentation to standard forms

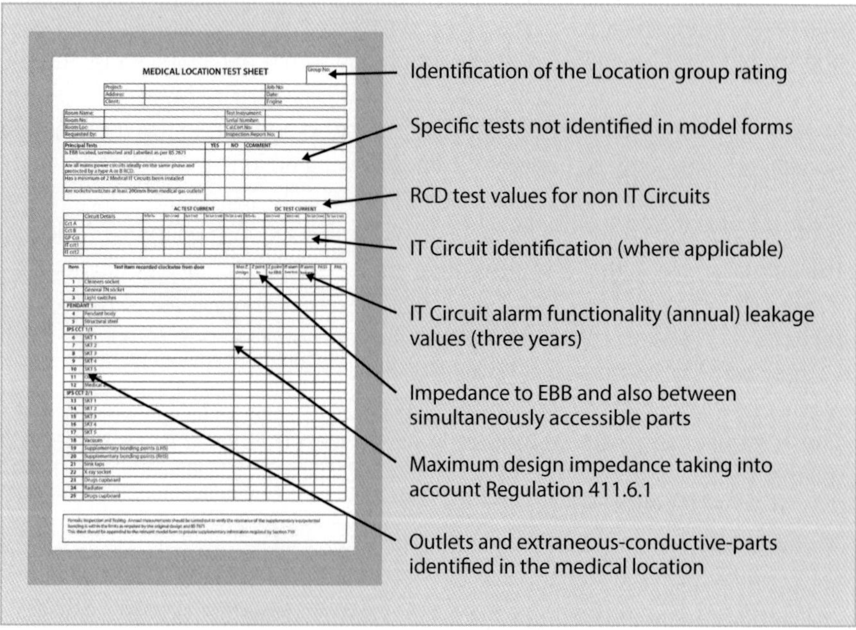

The aim of this form is to provide linking documentation between the IET model forms currently available to satisfy the general and the additional requirements set out in Section 710.

21.4 Colour of IT circuit conductors

HTM 06-01 advocates that output conductors from a medical IT transformer should both be brown as they are both live conductors not associated with earth.

A Guide to Electrical Installations in Medical Locations
© The Institution of Engineering and Technology

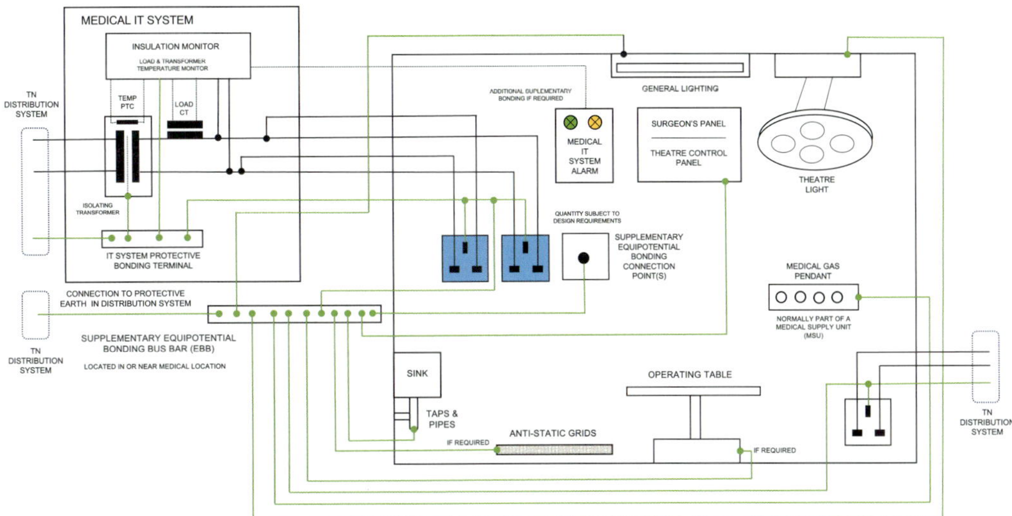

▼ **Figure 21.5** Indicative Group 2 theatre arrangement

Examining the 2007 version of HTM 06-01 further, it appears that this is not in line with Table 51 or other normative references in BS 7671. Figure 21.5 indicates the arrangement proposed for consideration in future editions of both HTM 06-01 and BS 7671 – currently, the HTM and group of documents and guidance based on or referencing the HTMs are the only documents that advocate this colour coding arrangement.

▼ **Table 21.2**   Table 51 of BS 7671

Function	Alphanumeric	Colour
Protective conductors		Green-and-yellow
Functional earthing conductor		Cream
AC power circuit [1]		
Line of single-phase circuit	L	Brown
Neutral of single- or three-phase circuit	N	Blue
Line 1 of three-phase AC circuit	L1	Brown
Line 2 of three-phase AC circuit	L2	Black
Line 3 of three-phase AC circuit	L3	Grey
Two-wire unearthed DC power circuit		
Positive of two-wire circuit	L+	Brown
Negative of two-wire circuit	L-	Grey
Two-wire earthed DC power circuit		
Positive (of negative earthed) circuit	L+	Brown
Negative (of negative earthed) circuit(2)	M	Blue
Positive (of positive earthed) circuit(2)	M	Blue

Negative (of positive earthed) circuit	L-	Grey
Three-wire DC power circuit		
Outer positive of two-wire circuit derived from three-wire system	L+	Brown
Outer negative of two-wire circuit derived from three-wire system	L-	Grey
Positive of three-wire circuit	L+	Brown
Mid-wire of three-wire circuit(2)(3)	M	Blue
Negative of three-wire circuit	L-	Grey
Control circuits, ELV and other applications		
Line conductor	L	Brown, Black, Red, Orange, Yellow, Violet, Grey, White, Pink or Turquoise
Neutral or mid-wire(4)	N or M	Blue

Neither of the conductors have reference to earth, so theoretically L1 and L2 may be brown as dictated by the 2007 version of HTM 06-01 and referenced in Chapter 9 of IET Guidance Note 7.

BS 7671 does not adopt the same approach for IT systems, with brown and blue cabling being set out in Table 51 of BS 7671 for AC systems. It should be noted that socket-outlets in medical IT circuits have a connection which states N for Neutral which suggests that there is a neutral, it is just not connected to earth. Designers should consider whether they wish to deviate from Table 51 of BS 7671 or follow the guidance set out in HTM 06-01 and Guidance Note 7. Although either method could be considered acceptable, common sense would dictate that the approach should be common throughout all medical IT system final circuits throughout the building/ development.

21.5 Testing ME equipment

Inspectors should be aware that all ME equipment connected to the electrical installation is outside the scope of BS 7671. Any testing of this ME equipment should therefore be carried out in accordance with BS EN 62353 and only performed by appropriately qualified personnel as indicated within BS EN 62353.

Imaging and diagnostics

22.1 General

There are very few visits to hospitals where the patient does not come into contact with imaging and diagnostics. Whilst some of the diagnostics will be part of a physical health assessment, for example, weight, height or respiration by way of pulse oximetry, and are carried out routinely, the demand for evidence and assurance of patient safety has led to increased use of other routine assessments such as the ECG. This demand has given rise to the provision of local equipment that is routinely used in wards and other areas.

22.2 Imaging-mains supply impedance

The mains supply impedance (both loop and line) must be sufficiently low to ensure that the disconnection times are achieved. What is sometimes overlooked is the need to meet possible lower impedances than would normally be expected for shock protection.

Where medical devices such as X-ray, CT and MR systems are installed it is essential to consult the manufacturers' documentation to ascertain the maximum mains supply line impedances. These systems often require very low phase-to-phase line impedances to meet the maximum power specifications of the equipment.

A typical 80 kW X-ray generator needs a phase-to-phase line impedance of 0.12 Ω or less at 400 V to achieve its rated maximum power at the nominal supply voltage. If the supply voltage was less, the maximum allowable line impedance is reduced, so in the previous example it would be 0.1 Ω at 360 V. If the line impedance is higher than allowed, the generators' maximum power would be reduced, which can lead to errors or poor diagnostic images due to increased exposure times (blurring then occurs as motion is not frozen).

In order to ensure that an X-ray generator can achieve its maximum rated power for X-ray exposures, it is important that the total line impedance is equal to, or lower than, the manufacturers' specified value. This depends on the design of the generator and its lowest working voltage needed to achieve maximum power.

Typical values are:

80 kW generator	380 V $\leq$ 0.1 Ω
80 kW generator	420 V $\leq$ 0.12 Ω
100 kW generator	380 V $\leq$ 0.08 Ω
100 kW generator	400 V $\leq$ 0.09 Ω

It can be seen that the lower the mains voltage, the lower the allowable line resistance becomes.

It should also be noted that these values are much lower than those needed to achieve the required disconnection times for protection.

22.3 Interventional X-ray systems and UPS

Permanently installed interventional X-ray systems are usually specified with a UPS in order to meet the requirements of IEC/BS EN 60601-2-43: *Particular requirements for the basic safety and essential performance of X-ray equipment for interventional procedures*. Clause 210.15.101 requires that the interventional X-ray equipment be placed in the cardiopulmonary resuscitation position (CPR) within 15 seconds. This is allowed to be increased by 1 s for each 15 ° of tilt the current working position deviates from the CPR position.

In order to meet this requirement a UPS is often specified to maintain the supply, only to the components that are essential; generally just the table and stand supplies. This is often referred to as the 'table-only option'. However, due to the type of procedures being performed, it may be essential to also maintain the ability to perform fluoroscopy during even very short mains failures.

This will of course require a larger UPS and associated batteries in order to enable this 'table and fluoroscopy only' solution, and may also be dependent upon machinery configuration.

Clinicians sometimes wish to be able to perform all procedures, including X-ray acquisitions, even during mains failures (no-break supply). This may be due to the complex nature of the case, as any break in supply may endanger the patient. This option is sometimes referred to as the 'full back-up option'.

The UPS systems for the machinery are generally not considered in HTM 06-01 (2007) tertiary power supplies. These UPS are being provided, in most cases, to meet the particular safety requirements of the ME equipment standard.

The autonomy of these UPS do not directly relate to any given time in Section 710, as normally the healthcare facility emergency supply will be available within 15 s. The autonomies in these instances relate to the medical equipment.

It should be noted that some systems may require a manual switchover from the UPS supply back to the normal mains supply and consideration needs to be given as to the period of time the UPS must be able to maintain. This will, to some extent, depend on the clinical requirements and possibly the available mains supply infrastructure.

In all the above cases it is essential to work with the clinicians and equipment manufacturers, including X-ray, UPS and control gear manufacturers, to ensure that the correct solution for their needs is properly identified and met.

22.4 Contactor control circuits

Many installations that involve medical imaging systems require the use of a contactor to switch the equipment power on and off, along with emergency power-off (STOP) buttons to be fitted.

This can cause some confusion about the wiring and operation of the contactor control and the location and type of emergency stop buttons to fit. Normally contactor control is only required for 3-phase equipment.

Some imaging equipment requires the mains power to be maintained, even with the medical imaging equipment switched off, in order to maintain the temperature of certain critical components. This can create an issue if mains power is lost through the night, as the imaging equipment may then take hours to warm up in the morning, delaying vital treatments. To prevent such an occurrence, the ME equipment manufacturer may specify special control systems to automatically restore the mains supply in the event of a power loss but only if it is safe to do so, for example, if none of the STOP switches have been operated. In such cases the installation instructions of the control equipment must be followed carefully.

22.4.1 Control circuit

▼ **Figure 22.1** Contactor control circuit

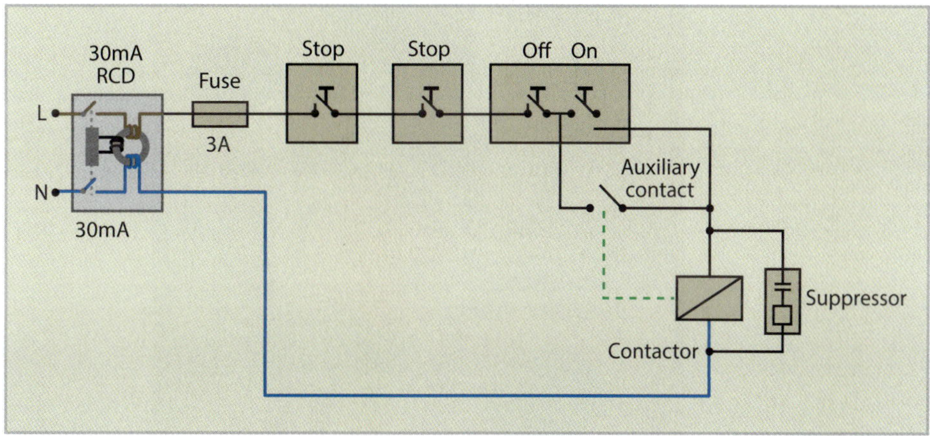

An RCD provides protection for the wiring, as required by Regulation 710.411.4, and a fuse for overcurrent protection. The contactor is fitted with a normally open auxiliary contact, which is used to maintain the supply to the contactor once the normally open ON button is pressed and released. If any of the STOP buttons or the OFF buttons are pressed, the supply is disconnected from the contactor and can't be re-established without pressing the ON button again, even if the STOP button is reset. The suppressor fitted across the contactor coil will prevent overvoltage and interference occurring when the supply to the coil is removed, increasing reliability and safety.

The contactor ON and OFF buttons should be marked with the standard international symbols for power ON and OFF.

Any indicator lamp for power on must be green or white in colour, not red, as this can cause confusion with previously described ME equipment standards for lamp colours. The use of long-life LEDs is suggested to aid reliability. It is also important to clearly mark the function of this control, for example, image equipment mains power.

22.4.2 STOP buttons

The selection and style of the STOP button is very important as this can affect the safety of the system.

A crucial point is that the unintentional operation of the STOP button must be avoided as, being in a medical location, continuity of supply is more than likely critical to safety. Consequently, only shrouded-style STOP buttons must be fitted and the use of locking buttons that require a key-switch to release them is not recommended, as this may delay the restoration of power if the key is misplaced.

It is also important to mark the function of any STOP buttons as it needs to be assured that users do not confuse these emergency mains supply power-off controls with any motion control stops mounted on the equipment that is used to prevent motorised movements but retains the power to the vital ME equipment.

▼ **Figure 22.2** Shrouded emergency stop buttons

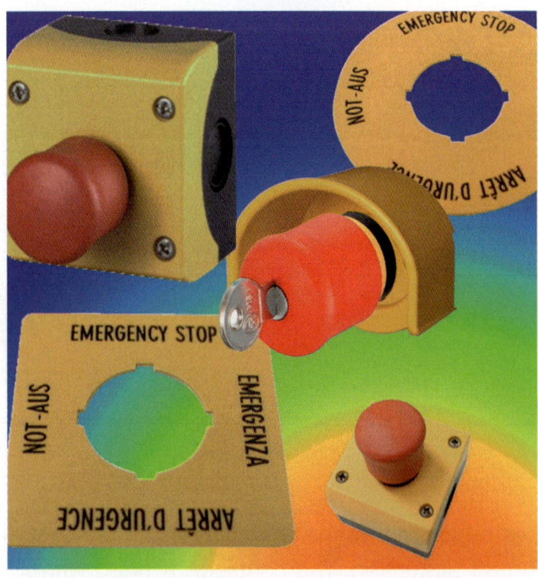

A sign should therefore be placed next to each emergency power-off STOP button with suitable wording, for example, 'Imaging Equipment Emergency Power Off'.

Normally, the ME equipment manufacturer will specify the location of any emergency power STOP buttons but it is normal to have a minimum of one in the examination room, which should be located where it is easily visible but not likely to be accidentally operated.

It is also essential to provide one in a room where the ME equipment control cabinets are located, separate from the examination equipment, so that service personnel can operate in an emergency. One may also be required in the control room if the contactor control (ON/OFF) is not easily visible or accessible. Where the ME equipment control cabinets are located in a separate room from the examination equipment, a remote contactor control (ON/OFF) may be required for ease of service.

22.5 Illuminated warning signs

Some ME equipment may require the installation of illuminated warning signs on the entrance doors to certain medical locations to inform users of potentially dangerous conditions, such as the use of X-rays or lasers. The location and style of these illuminated signs is normally specified by the design engineer following the expert advice of the local radiation protection advisor (RPA) who is the appointed person responsible for radiological matters.

These illumined warning signs may be supplied from the ME equipment or by a wall switch as part of the electrical installation enabling works. They may be low voltage (24 V) or, more normally, 230 V mains. Where the equipment is Class I, the earth for the sign would normally be connected to the EBB.

All X-ray installations will require illuminated warning signs in order to comply with the Ionising Radiation Regulations 1999, which the RPA would advise upon. Because the radiation is often of short duration and rapid frequency, care needs to be taken when selecting lamps used for these signs.

Traditionally, standard incandescent lamps have been used in illuminated warning signs, rather than fluorescent lamps. In line with various technological changes and the move towards the use of LED technology, some signs are now being supplied with LED emitters.

Although LED lighting is attractive due to its intensity and low energy usage, care should be taken in unit and relay selection. Anecdotal evidence suggests that some designs may not be suitable for the rapid switching that can be expected in certain imaging procedures, for example, guided fluoroscopy. Consequently, any design using a switch-mode power supply to drive the LEDs may, in some cases, be unsuitable, since the high in-rush currents that switch-mode power supplies exhibit during rapid switching will cause the standard control relay contacts to weld together. This high in-rush current is multiplied by the number of signs connected together in parallel, as dictated by the number of entrances to be protected, which further increase the chances of a control relay failure.

It is therefore important to confirm with the illuminated sign supplier that any sign can cope with the rapid switching on and off that can be expected with X-ray systems, especially those for CT, fluoroscopy and interventional medical systems.

Often, an illuminated warning sign is needed to indicate a controlled area. These signs normally illuminate when the ME equipment is switched on and go out only when the ME equipment is switched off. Sometimes, depending on local requirements, the sign is required to be illuminated when the mains supply to the equipment is energised. In such cases, the electrical enabling works need to make provision for this supply. However, it is important that, when the same sign contains two lights, one for 'Controlled Area' and another for X-ray or laser 'On', the supply for the two sections remains isolated from each other.

Historic guidance documents such as MEIGaN demanded that the control circuits be on the same phase as each other. When managing circuits, this might be sensible, however, if two phases or two separate circuits are provided, suitable warning and details for the maintainer should also be provided to prevent danger.

Use of red light

The use of a red light is normally not allowed within the patient environment in order to meet the requirements of BS EN 60601-1. However, the use of red lights to restrict entry is normal practice, since they are located outside the patient environment and mostly outside any Group 1 or Group 2 medical location.

Mobile medical locations

23

Traditionally, these have been single purpose vehicles, for example, mammography units that were used to supply services in different areas where either there was no facility or to provide additional facilities to meet demand.

Mobile surgical units have been traditionally used to treat wounded service personnel, providing lifesaving support and other treatment. However, there are now a number of healthcare providers utilising mobile surgical and diagnostic facilities to treat NHS patients.

An example of this at the time of publication there is an NHS service provision by the private sector provider that runs throughout the former Greater Manchester area and that operates a mobile assessment and treatment service using a number of articulated lorry-based mobile facilities. These units are comprised of a minimum of five trailers, which are connected together to provide assessment and treatment services, including:

(a) consultation with a specialist following GP referral:
(b) physical health measurements and ECGs;
(c) diagnostics in terms of X-ray, CT and MRI;
(d) treatment in terms of medical interventions; and
(e) surgical interventions such as lumps and bumps removal, vasectomy, etc.

These units, when connected together, form the mobile clinic and hospital outpatient department. The units are self-powered and are totally independent of the electricity supply due to a generator unit that powers the mobile units. These generators are specifically designed to power the units and are fitted with a UPS that helps to smooth out any significant demand in the unit. The picture in Figure 23.1 indicate the five-vehicle hook-up. The generator vehicle being located to the rear 'ancillary' side of the hook up arrangement out of view of the public.

▼ **Figure 23.1** Mobile medical locations (image courtesy of North West CATS)

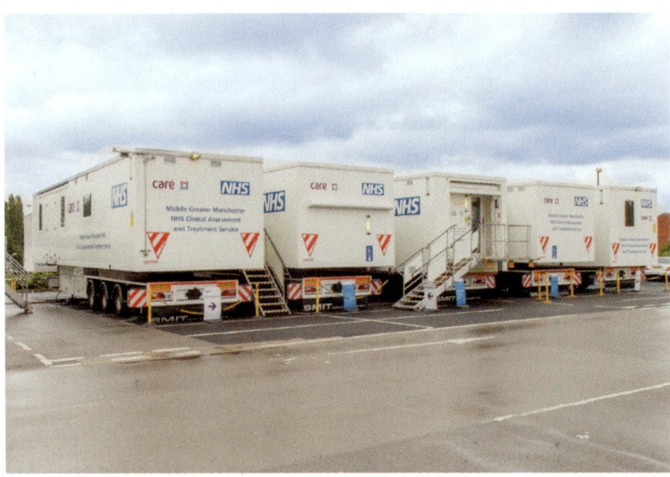

In this service provision, the units are supplied from a bespoke, independent generator and UPS configuration, some of the normal pitfalls experienced by similar mobile units are avoided. In this instance they have had to overcome overnight challenges such as noise pollution etc. as no regular mains supply is available.

Regardless of the function or the nature of how electricity is supplied, it should be remembered that mobile medical locations are subject to the requirements of BS 7671 in a number of ways.

The designer of the installation needs to therefore take into account the requirements of more than one special location, i.e. Section 710 and Section 717.

Appendix

Information supporting medical location assessment

1

▼ **Table A.1** Annex 710 from BS 7671

Medical location	Group			Classification	
	0	1	2	≤ 0.5 s	> 0.5 s ≤ 15 s
1 Massage room	X	X			X
2 Bedrooms		X			X
3 Delivery room		X		X[a]	X
4 ECG, EEG, EHG room		X			X
5 Endoscopic room		X[b]		X	X[b]
6 Examination or treatment room		X		X	X
7 Urology room		X[b]		X	X[b]
8 Radiological diagnostic and therapy room		X	X	X	X
9 Hydrotherapy room		X			X
10 Physiotherapy room		X			X
11 Anaesthetic area			X	X[a]	X
12 Operating theatre			X	X[a]	X
13 Operating preparation room			X	X[a]	X
14 Operating plaster room			X	X[a]	X
15 Operating recovery room			X	X[a]	X
16 Heart catheterization room			X	X[a]	X
17 Intensive care room			X	X[a]	X
18 Angiographic examination room			X	X[a]	X
19 Haemodialysis room		X			X
20 Magnetic resonance imaging (MRI) room		X	X	X	X
21 Nuclear medicine		X			X
22 Premature baby room			X	X[a]	X
23 Intermediate Care Unit (IMCU)			X	X	X

a   Luminaires and life-support medical electrical equipment which needs power supply within 0.5 s or less.
b   Not being an operating theatre.

▼ **Table A.2** Classification of safety services for medical locations

Classification	Change over times (seconds)	Description of classification
No break	0	Automatic supply available at no-break
Very short break	0.15	Automatic supply available within 0.15 s
Short break	0.5	Automatic supply available within 0.5 s
Medium break	15	Automatic supply available within 15 s
Long break	>15	Automatic supply available in more than 15 s

Note:

1 Generally it is unnecessary to provide a no-break power supply for ME equipment. However, certain microprocessor controlled equipment may require such a supply.

2 Safety services provided for locations having differing classifications should meet that classification which gives the highest security of supply.

A2.1 Myth 1: the purpose of an IPS is to protect the patient from 'microshocks'

There is a misunderstanding in the industry that a medical IT system, also known as an isolated power supply (IPS), is provided to protect the patient from 'microshocks'.

Shock hazards due to bodily contact with the 50 Hz mains supply are well known and documented. These findings are listed in IEC/TR2 60479-1 *Effects of current on human beings and livestock – general aspects.*

According to BS EN 60601, patient leakage currents of the order of 10 µA have a probability of 0.2 % for causing ventricular fibrillation or pump failure when applied through a small area of the heart. At 50 µA (microshock), the probability of ventricular fibrillation increases to 1 %.

If we examine an isolation transformer that is compliant with BS EN 61558-2-15, we will see that there is no galvanic connection between the primary and the secondary windings.

▼ **Figure A2.1** Isolation transformer arrangement

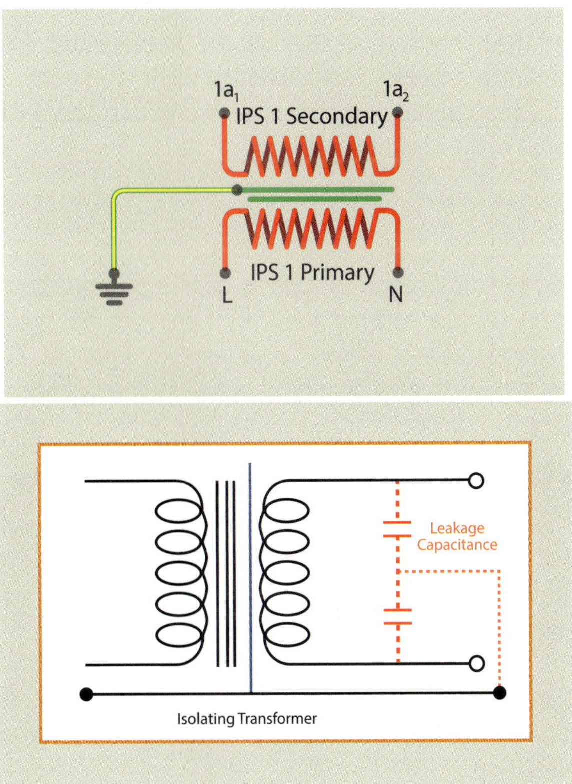

However, due to capacitive coupling on the secondary winding, there will be small currents flowing. As a result, instead of the scenario in (a), due to compromised patients the situation is more likely to be that of (b). However, this is unrealistic as a patient should not come into direct contact with live parts as medical electrical equipment to BS 60601 is used.

▼ **Figure A2.2** IT system hazards

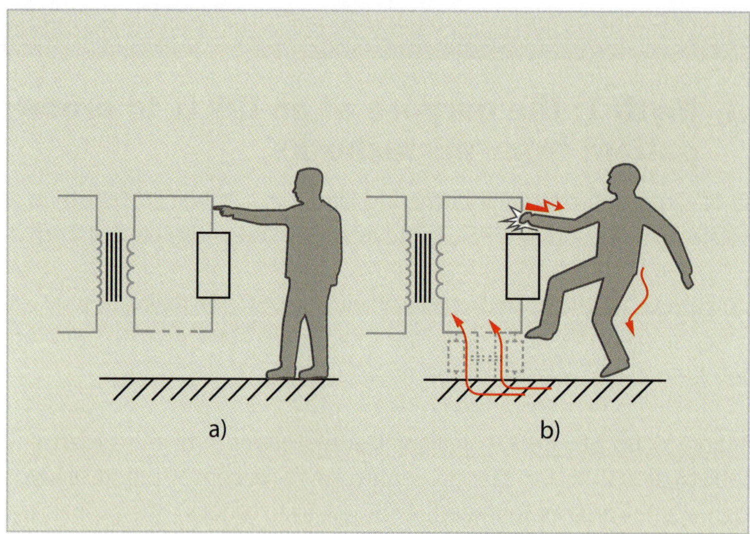

Consequently, this system will not protect the patient from 'microshocks'. That is the purpose of medical electrical equipment. The medical IT system is provided to give first fault to earth resilience and warnings. Examples of the use of this type of protection can be seen where a patient's drink or fluid is spilled on the ME equipment; instead of causing a fault that trips the local circuit-breaker, the system detects an earth fault as the impedance of the equipment falls below the threshold and sounds the alarm.

This gives staff the opportunity to seek out the problem and, if appropriate, unplug the equipment or obtain a replacement. Although there is an earth fault, the IT element of the system is compromised and, should a second fault (on a different polarity) occur, this would result in the loss of supply.

In summary:

As the isolated electrical supply provides a degree of protection against electric shock for fully dressed, healthy patients, the IT system does not provide protection against the low level 'microshocks' that can cause harm to a patient. The primary purpose of a medical IT system is to provide a level of first fault resilience.

A2.2 Myth 2: medical locations should be single phase

The original intent of MEIGaN (now withdrawn) was to provide support to those installing new imaging equipment installations in poorly maintained, out-of-date hospitals with wiring systems that were equally out of date and contained faults on the existing circuits.

This created an approach that was potentially overly cautious. These documents also only focused on a single installation that would typically be a modification or extension of a department.

There have, for a number of years, been considerable changes in NHS diagnostics and treatment, coupled with an investment in healthcare premises generally. The investment has created large-scale projects and developments so that now, instead of adding one item on to the end of a unit, a new suite of theatres or diagnostic areas are created with supporting beds to meet demand. The funding has also brought about considerable changes to estates, some of which were bogged down in backlog maintenance.

One of the limitations set down in early guidance was the requirement that all installations be single phase. This is based on the misconception that, as circuits were on different phases, there would be, for some reason, a 400 V touch voltage between equipment.

A great deal of concern exists in Group 2 medical locations, particularly about socket-outlets in the patient environment. When examining medical IT systems, a number of observations can be made. Firstly, there is no galvanic connection between medical IT circuits and/or TN circuits, and no connection between different IT circuits from different medical IT systems (here in the figures, the references are 'IPS' for brevity and convenience instead of 'medical IT system').

▼ **Figure A2.3** Medical IT transformers supplied from same and different phases

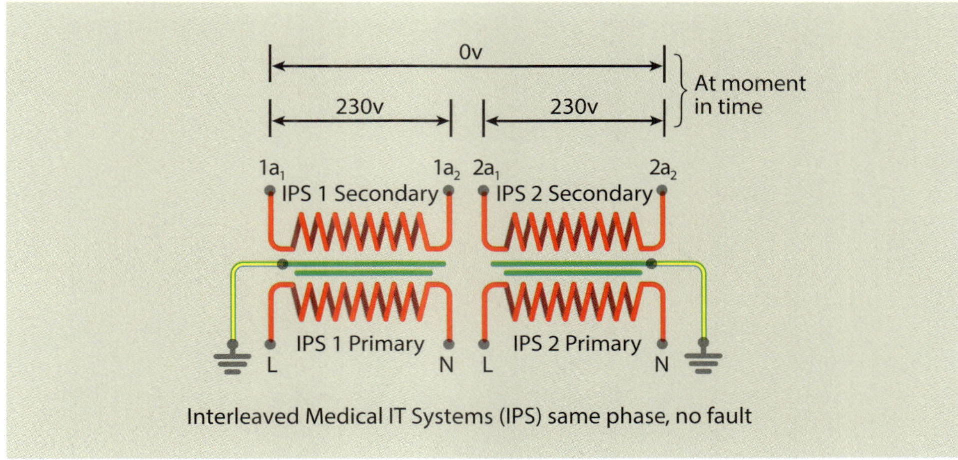

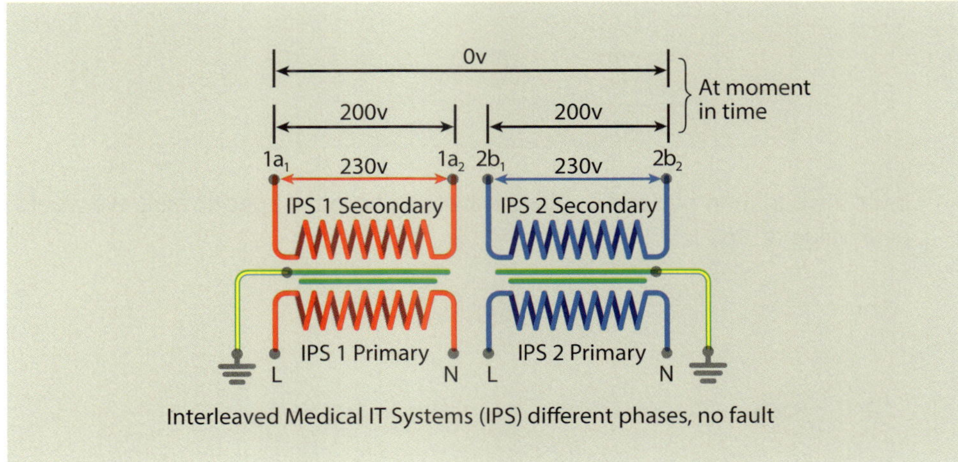

It can be seen that, at a specific moment in time, the voltages between the two different IT systems remain at 0 V across the live conductors while the voltage across the live terminals $1a_1$ to $1a_2$ and $2a_1$ and $2a_2$ will be 230 V. As these are isolation transformers to BS EN 61558-2-15, the voltage between live conductors and earth will be 0 V as there is no connectivity or reference to earth.

▼ **Figure A2.4** Fault on IT transformer secondary circuits — same phase

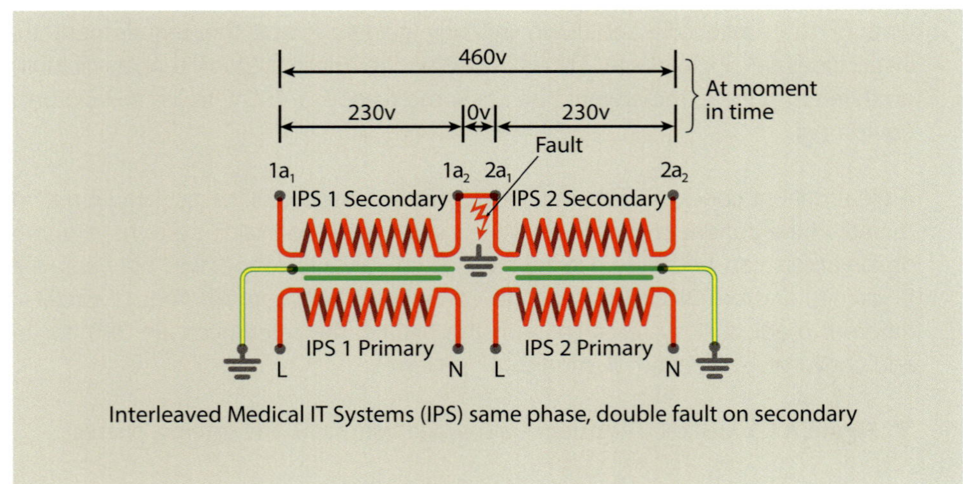

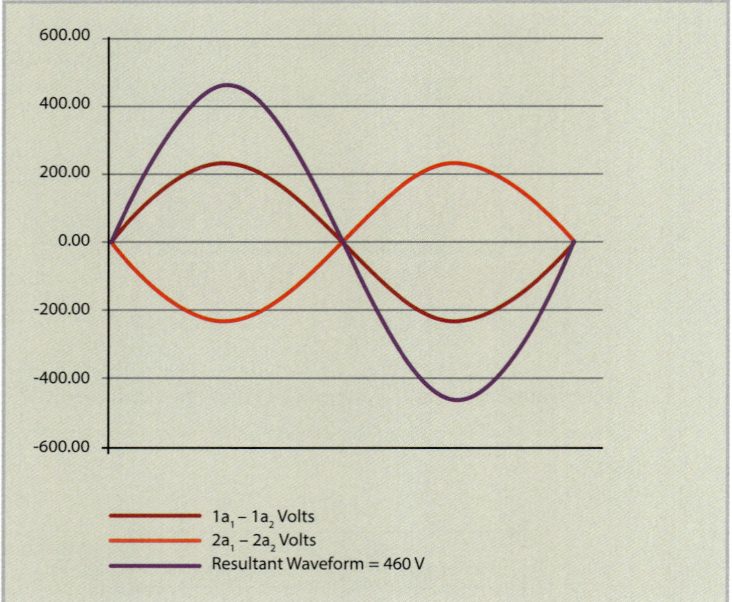

If we were to then plot the resulting waveform from the specific fault, we would get a peak value of 460 V.

A Guide to Electrical Installations in Medical Locations
© The Institution of Engineering and Technology

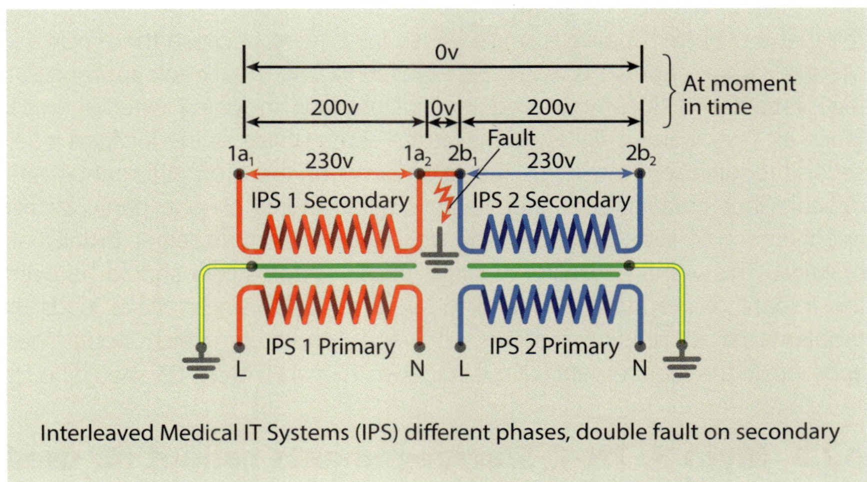

▼ **Figure A2.5** Fault on IT transformer secondary circuits — different phases

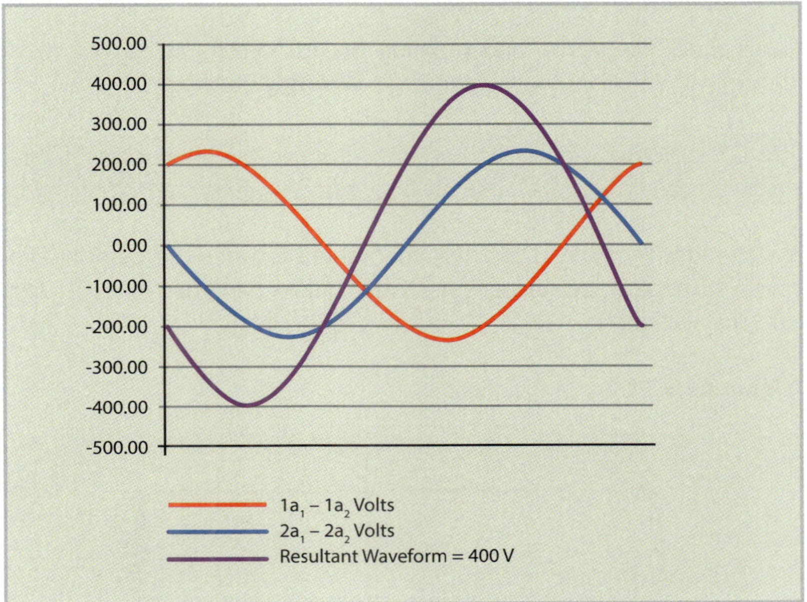

If we look at the identical fault between medical IT systems that are fed from different phases and plot the resulting waveform from the specific fault, we would get a peak value of 400 V.

In terms of medical locations, there is no reason why correctly installed single-phase systems are safer than polyphase systems. There is no known effect on the patients, the equipment is not affected by being on different phases and it certainly does not deviate from BS 7671. However, HTM 08-03 which relates to bedhead services does require all supplies in a room to be on the same phase.

Anecdotally, in the region of 50 % of the installation contractors, and a larger number of consulting engineers, believe that socket-outlets on different phases in the same room was in fact a deviation from the general requirements of BS 7671.

A2.2.1 Subjective selection

Historically the reason for a single-phase system is to two-fold. Firstly, the designer has felt that it is better to have a single-phase installation because there was a belief that there is a risk that persons would be exposed to 400 V between appliances. Secondly, legacy guidance documents required installations including external warning lights (such as X-ray warning lights) to be on the same phase as the location it served. The second requirement means demarcation between areas on different phases became difficult, thus creating large areas across departments on one particular phase. This arrangement of large areas on one phase, particularly in larger installations, is not practical. This irrational feeling of single-phase systems only should be overcome for the benefit of the installation and to avoid unwieldy single-phase loads that create problems for distribution systems, UPS and generators, which would mean where appropriate the requirement set out in Clause 7.12 of HTM 08-03 should be challenged.

A2.3 Myth 3: TN-C-S arrangements cannot be used in medical locations

There is much discussion and mention of TNS circuits in existing medical location guidance, with MEIGaN (now withdrawn) **wrongly** stating that:

> *"A TN-C-S system is one in which earth and neutral are common over part of the system. In many cases this arises due to a fault in some remote location…"*

This statement is incorrect and has contributed towards the demonisation of TN-C-S supplies in medical locations. Protective multiple earthing (PME) is designated as a TN-C-S installation.

▼ **Figure A2.6** TN-C-S arrangement

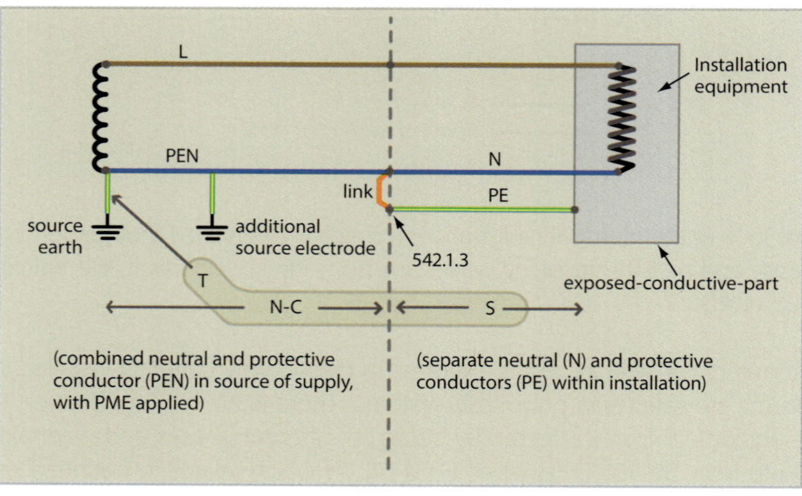

TN-C-S is an internationally recognised method of earthing. It is the prominent form of LV arrangement in urban areas of the UK and is used in millions of dwellings and non-residential installations.

> **Note:** Where a supply is from the public low voltage distribution system, regardless of the apparent connection arrangement at the consumer intake position, the arrangement may still be connected to a PME system.

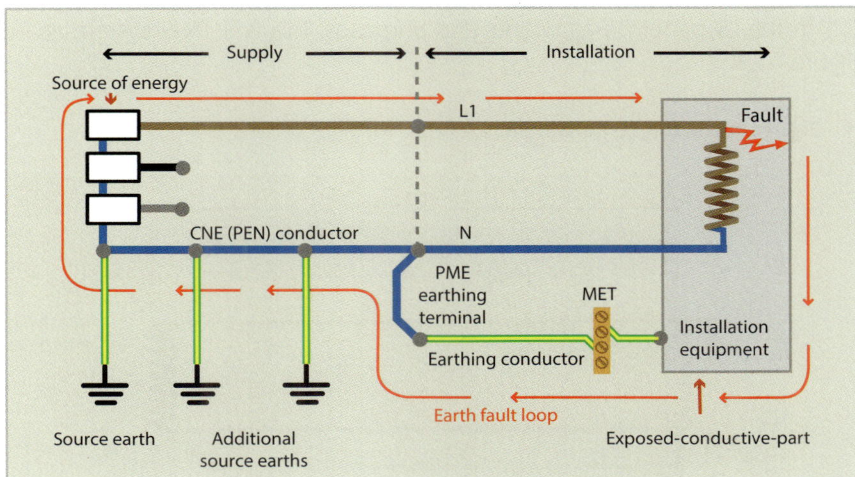

▼ **Figure A2.7** PME arrangement

It should be recognised that PME has its own limitations, which includes restrictions on use in areas such as petrol stations, caravan pitch supplies and restrictions on use of galvanically connected external water taps. This is because, in the unlikely event of loss of neutral, a loss in earth path may occur. This very low probability has virtually no consequence to those within the bonded environment.

However, there are obvious instances where residual dangers are present that could result in lethal voltages. For example, an external metal tap, earthed through the PME system, with a potential for a wet connection with true Earth. An example of a different but wider reaching potential to cause harm would be that of a petrol filling station where, through loss of the system earth, the fuel tanks and pipework could become a secondary conductor/earth electrode. A final example is that of a person outside the equipotential zone, in contact with true Earth when the neutral that provides the earthing conductor is potentially live as a result of the discontinuity of the neutral conductor, which will effectively make the system earth and all that is connected to it live.

As a result of such potential dangers, PMEs are forbidden in caravans and restricted in mobile or transportable units.

The designation TN-C-S does not always mean that the supply is a PME supply, however; often, a private transformer uses a TN-C-S arrangement to the neutral earth link in the LV panel. To all intents and purposes, this is a TN-S system as indicated in Figure A2.8.

▼ **Figure A2.8** TN-S arrangement

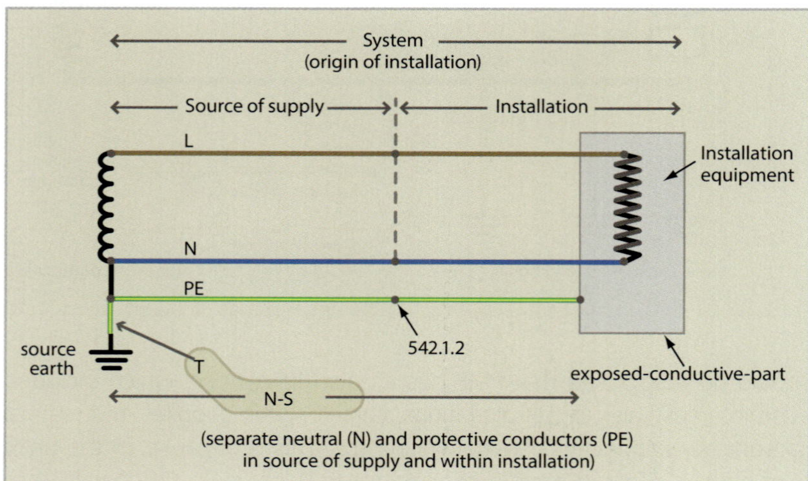

Note: In a TN-S system, there has to be a neutral earth link at some point; this is the very nature of TN systems.

Looking at the reasoning as to why this myth has come about, it is likely that there has been confusion of the TN-C-S and TN-C systems. Unlike TN-C-S, TN-C is not permitted in the UK.

Regulation 710.312.2 of BS 7671 states that "PEN conductors shall not be used in medical locations and medical buildings downstream of the main distribution board". This is further qualified by the note that states: "In Great Britain Regulation 8(4) of the Electricity Safety, Quality and Continuity Regulations prohibits the use of PEN conductors in consumers' installations".

In summary, TN-C-S installations are not prohibited in medical locations unless that location is a mobile or a transportable unit, as there is no reason why a PME supply cannot be used to supply an indoor, fixed medical location. This has been recently clarified at IEC committee level recognising the danger as being a PEN conductor arrangement in the installation and not a PME installation.

A2.4 Myth 4: Group 2 medical locations touch voltages should be less than 10 mV

Research shows that a current of 10 µA flowing through small areas inside the heart has a 0.2 % chance of causing ventricular fibrillation in a patient, which is about the same as the effect from mechanical stimulation by the tip of a catheter in the heart.

Historically, some guidance documents, such as MEIGaN (now withdrawn), have taken this 10 µA value and applied the human body resistance of 1 kΩ to come up with a 10 mV limit for measuring touch voltage between accessible conductive parts of the electrical installation. However, this approach is fundamentally flawed.

The electrical installation should never come into direct contact with the heart. If this were so, the entire electrical installation would need to meet the medical device directive and all parts of BS EN 60601 would apply, which would be a costly and onerous, if not impossible, task.

This value of 10 µA is correctly used within BS EN 60601-1 as the limit value for CF applied parts when the medical device is in 'normal' condition. CF applied parts are parts of the ME equipment that could come into direct contact with the heart. In fault conditions, such as the protective earth conductor becoming disconnected, BS EN 60601-1 allows the CF applied parts leakage current limit of 50 µA. This is why some documents refer to a touch voltage of 50 mV, as they have taken this 'worst case' limit as their guide.

One other point to note is that the 'F' used in 'BF' and 'CF' applied parts refers to parts that are floating or isolated from earth, with additional protective measures applied to CF parts over BF. Since the historic measurement of touch voltages are always measured between earth connections, it is clear that these 'F' type limits are completely inappropriate.

Figure A2.9 gives the limit values for the main types of applied parts.

▼ **Figure A2.9** Main types of applied part summary of permitted leakage

Symbol	Applied part type	Definition/description	Normal Condition (NC)	Single Fault Condition (SFC)
	Type B Applied Part	**TYPE B APPLIED PART** APPLIED PART complying with the specified requirements of BS EN 60601 to provide protection against electric shock, particularly regarding allowable PATIENT LEAKAGE CURRENT and PATIENT AUXILIARY CURRENT	100µA	500µA
	Type BF Applied Part	**TYPE BF APPLIED PART** F-TYPE APPLIED PART complying with the specified requirements of BS EN 60601 to provide a higher degree of protection against electric shock than that provided by TYPE B APPLIED PARTS	100µA	500µA
	Type CF Applied Part	**TYPE CF APPLIED PART** F-TYPE APPLIED PART complying with the specified requirements BS EN 60601 to provide a higher degree of protection against electric shock than that provided by TYPE BF APPLIED PARTS	10µA	50µA

The above values are for a.c. current and for a single applied part only. Other values exist for d.c. and multiple applied parts.

Figure A2.10 is provided in order to give an indication of the level of isolation required to achieve an F-type applied part.

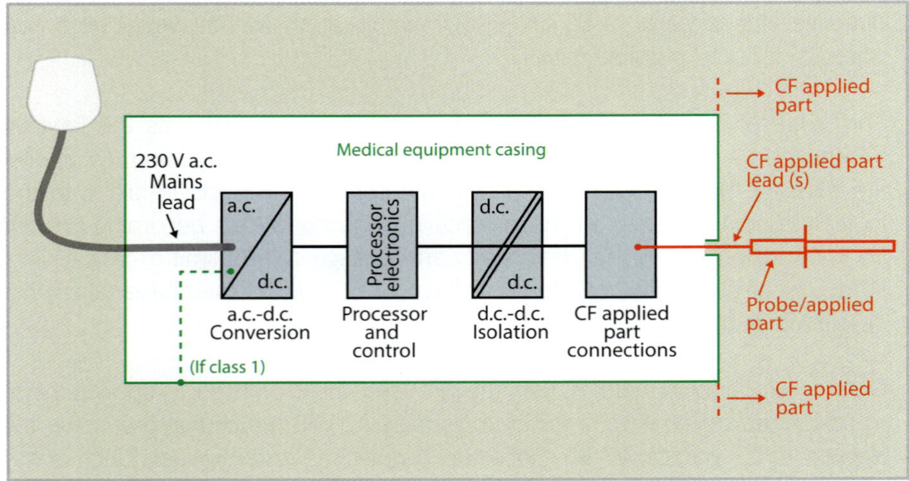

▼ **Figure A2.10** CF applied part isolation

The closest we could get to finding a value from BS EN 60601-1 that could in any way be used with reference to the electrical installation is the value for touch leakage current, which was known as 'enclosure leakage current' in previous editions.

▼ **Figure A2.11** Touch leakage

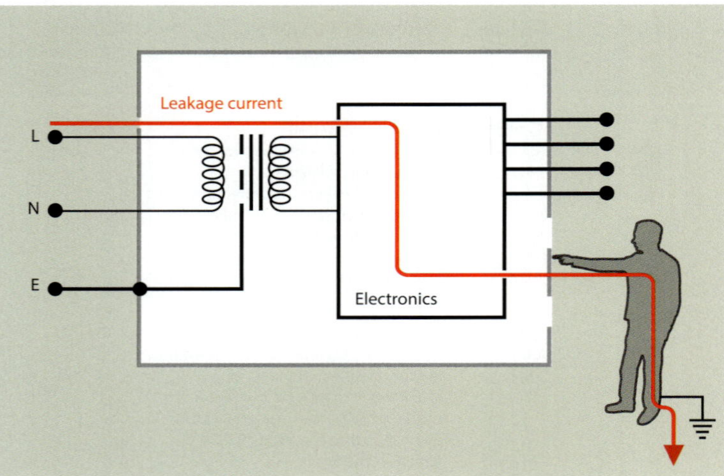

This touch leakage current is defined as: "leakage current flowing from the enclosure or from parts thereof, excluding patient connections, accessible to any operator or patient in normal use, through an external path, other than the protective earth conductor to earth or to another part of the enclosure." This can also be current induced into conductive parts that are not connected to earth, which could, for example, equate to touching Class II equipment.

The limit is set to the same values as those for B-type applied parts: 100 μA in normal conditions and 500 μA in single fault conditions. These values are still considered safe due to the low probability of the operator incorrectly handling an intra-cardiac catheter at the same time as touching the enclosure of the ME equipment.

However, since we can't 'unplug' the entire Group 2 medical location and place it on a test bench to perform the measurements as mandated by BS EN 60601, it is pointless to try to meet any of these requirements. In fact, the measurements of 10 mV, 50 mV or 100 mV using standard high impedance digital volt-meter (DVM) is futile, as often parts that are isolated from earth can have very high potentials that will collapse to nothing when loaded with human body contact. This has often caused engineering staff to chase 'ghost' values, creating unnecessary work.

If all the requirements of BS 7671 are fully and correctly applied, the risk of any voltages, however small, occurring between any of the protective parts or extraneous-conductive-parts is negligible for the reduced touch voltage (25 V AC 60 V DC) requirements of the location in normal conditions and fault conditions.

Figure A2.12 below shows an intra-cardiac procedure indicating the potential for any patient leakage and the irrelevance of touch voltages in the location with respect to the patient and the environment.

▼ **Figure A2.12** Intra-cardiac procedure using CF rated equipment

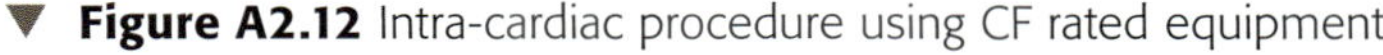

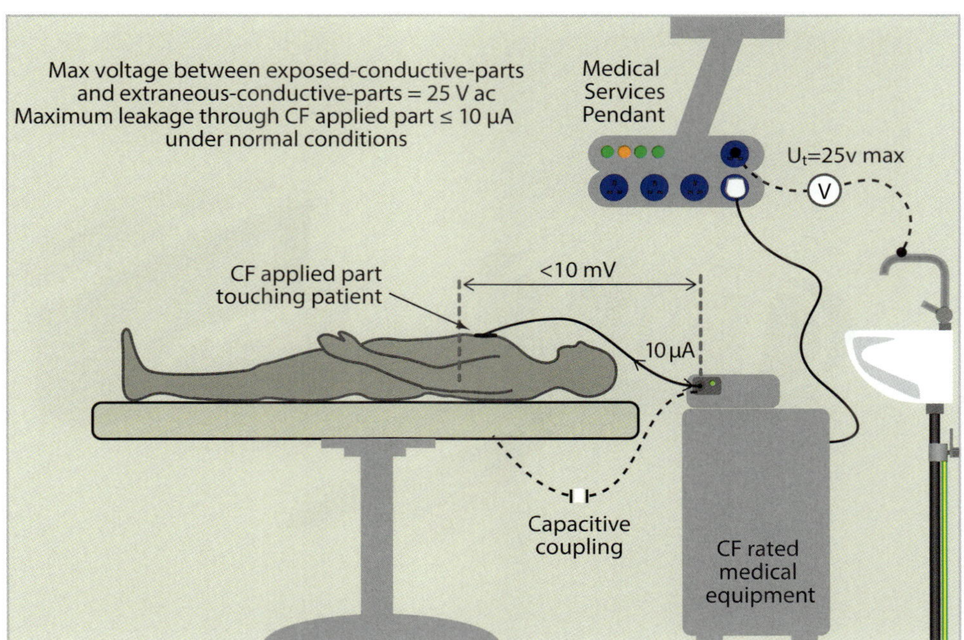

The electrical installation should never come into direct contact with the heart. The possibility of an operator directly touching a catheter at the same time as touching a part of the electrical installation (via the earth of some ME equipment) is very low, as this is extremely bad practice.

Note: Operator would be gloved which again would provide a further level of resistance into any theoretical scenario.

A2.5 Myth 5: sensor taps in Group 2 medical locations

There is still a culture of checking for touch voltages using a high impedance digital voltmeter (DVM). It is possible through random testing with high impedance DVMs that various voltage readings will be observed on metalwork in any location, however, due to historic guidance documents, it is usual for this type of test to be carried out in a Group 2 medical location.

The main reason for these random voltages will normally be small induced voltages that are picked up by the metalwork.

There have been various reports of voltages that are much higher than the standard touch voltage of 25 V AC, even when no fault is evident. This has previously been blamed on long-term overloads to earth that have not been cleared by the protective device. Whilst this is not impossible, it is highly unlikely due to the level of protective bonding that is installed in an ordinary installation that does not have the level of supplementary equipotential bonding found in a Group 1 or Group 2 medical location.

▼ **Figure A2.13** Typical test instruments (image courtesy of Megger Limited)

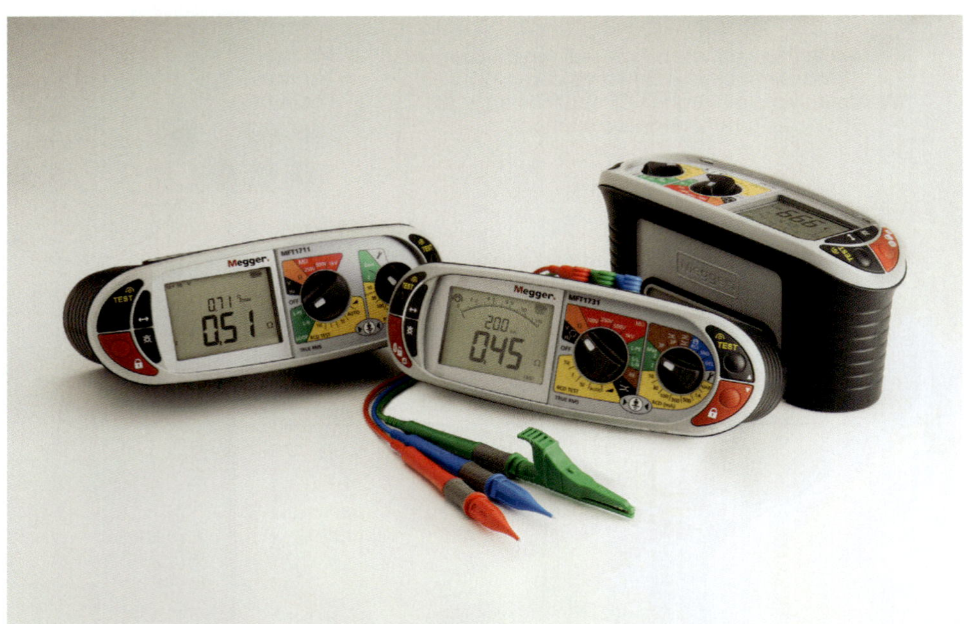

When investigating reports of dangerous touch voltages, it can often be seen that the reports usually relate to Class II equipment. This is linked to the phenomena whereby when certain types of Class II equipment are powered up, a perceived voltage can be detected on the Class II metalwork.

Reports received have been from 30 V to a maximum of 80 V. Examining the phenomena, we can see that Class II equipment will have a level of capacitive coupling and, theoretically, with the capacitive coupling on a TN system it is possible that 115 V is being induced onto the metalwork, as indicated below.

▼ **Figure A2.14** Theoretical voltage value due to capacitive coupling

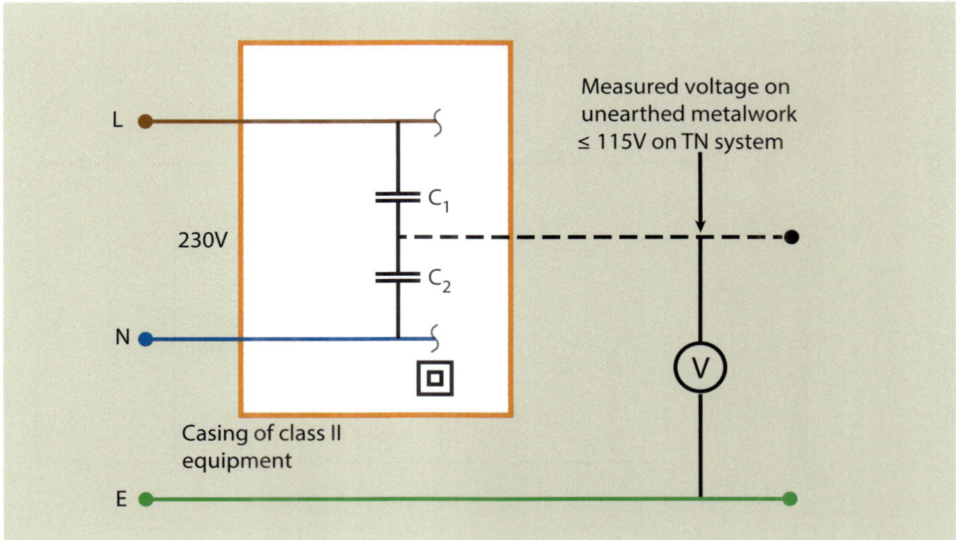

Capacitive coupling provides a theoretical maximum induced voltage of 115 V. However, the maximum value will not be read due to the current demand of the high impedance DVM, for example, the higher the impedance the nearer the value to the theoretical value.

This scenario is not dangerous on a non-faulty installation. In order to check the voltage is strictly due to capacitive coupling the human body equivalent circuit or the IEC 60601 filter should be used, as shown in Figure A2.15.

▼ **Figure A2.15** The human body equivalent circuit or IEC 60601 filter

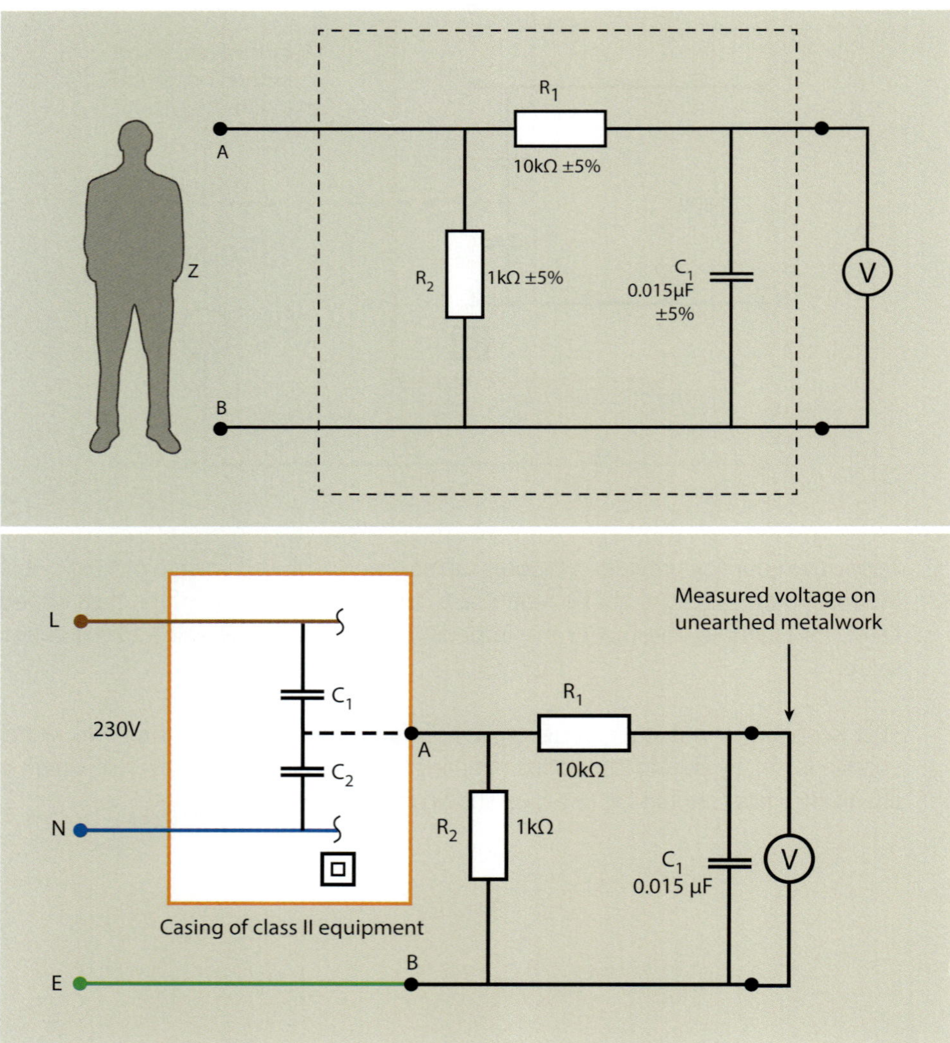

By adding the human body equivalent circuit to test measurements, voltages previously measured as being excessive have fallen to virtually zero. Provided that supplementary equipotential bonding is in place, there is no need to provide additional bonding to taps that are fed from a Class II valve. This test often removes the need for additional supplementary equipotential bonding and removes the erroneous test results that can result in engineers chasing 'ghost' values of touch voltages.

Appendix 3
Generator fault levels

A3.1 Generator fault levels

The public supply network has a huge generating infrastructure behind it to deliver electricity across the UK. Whilst different parts of the network have considerably different characteristics due to location etc., it would be reasonable to assume that the mains supply would have a larger prospective fault level than a reciprocating diesel engine set.

Although this assumption may be correct in principle, throughout the initial period of a long-term fault supplied by a generator, a number of different phenomena occur. The generator has a number of time-related characteristics to consider, starting from the initial moment of fault, through the period affected by sub-transient reactance, through the transient and ultimately into the synchronous characteristics of the machine output and its impact on installation calculations.

▼ **Figure A3.1** Initial symmetrical short circuit

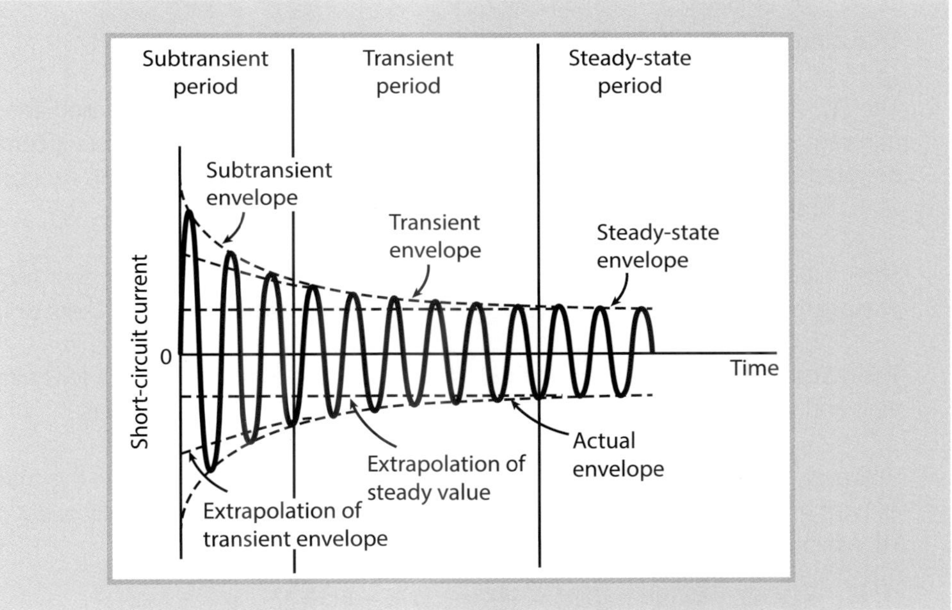

A3.1.1 Initial fault online calculations

With a generator operating at full voltage, a symmetrical 3-phase short circuit at its terminals will cause a large amount of current to flow.

Generator direct axis sub-transient reactance X"d is the reactance of the stator winding at the instance of fault.

The initial instantaneous current value $\mathrm{ISC_{sym}}$ is controlled by the sub-transient reactance X"d and is expressed as follows:

$$I\,"\,SC_{sym} = E_{AC} \div X\,"_d$$

or using the per unit method:

$$I\,"\,SC_{sym} = I_{flc} \div X\,"_d PU$$

where:

$I"SC_{sym}$ is the sub-transient symmetrical short circuit current.

I_{FLC} is machine full load current, measured in Amps.

$X"d$ is generator direct axis sub-transient reactance, per unit.

Typically, the values of generator reactances are published per unit on a specified base alternator rating, and are therefore likely to be shown as per unit values. It should be noted that many per unit values have a tolerance in the order of 10 %, which should be included when considering worst case scenarios.

The base needs no adjustment for the purpose of our calculations.

Example: a 400 V, 1000 kVA, 800 kW generator has a transient reactance (X") of 10.1 % or 0.101 PU or, worst case, could be 0.101 pu −10 % = 0.091PU.

The initial fault current would be:

$$I_{flc} = kVA \text{ rating} \div (V_{1\text{-}1} \times \sqrt{3}) = 1443\ A$$

$$I\,"SC_{sym} = 1443 \div 0.091 = 15857\ A$$

This is considerably larger than the 1,443 A full-load current.

The AC flowing in the generator during the sub-transient period is called the sub-transient current and is denoted by I". The time constant of the sub-transient current is denoted by T" and it can be determined from the slope. This current can be as much as 10 times the full-load fault current.

This initial symmetrical short-circuit current is used to determine the required prospective short-circuit current rating of overcurrent devices, circuit-breakers or fuses.

This value is the limiting factor in the first 5 to 6 cycles or the first 0.12 s following the fault and is likely to operate the instantaneous settings on circuit-breakers.

However, this is not the end of the process as there are more changes to the machine as time goes on. If we look further on in the direction of the fault we will see X'd and Xd, which are 19.6 % or .196 PU and 350 % or 3.5 PU, worst case.

$$I\,'SC_{sym} = 1443 \div (0.196 - 10\%) = 1443 \div 0.176 = 8198\ A$$

The current I' is in the order of 5 times the full-load fault current.

Following the transient period, the synchronous reactance takes effect:

$$I^{ss}\,SC_{sym} = 1443 \div (3.5 - 10\%) = 1443 \div 3.15 = 412\ A$$

In this instance, the steady state fault current is approximately one third the normal full-load rating.

▼ **Figure A3.2** Generator output over the three stages

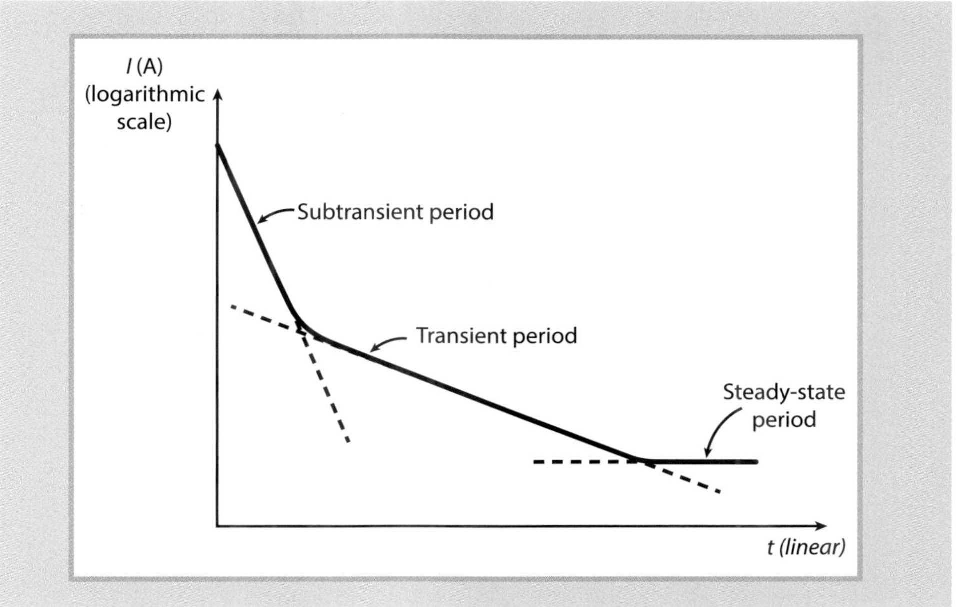

As can be seen, in this period the fault level is approximately one third of the normal full load delivery.

This can vary from machine to machine and depends on the type of excitation.

▼ **Figure A3.3** Effect of excitation (image courtesy of Schneider Electric)

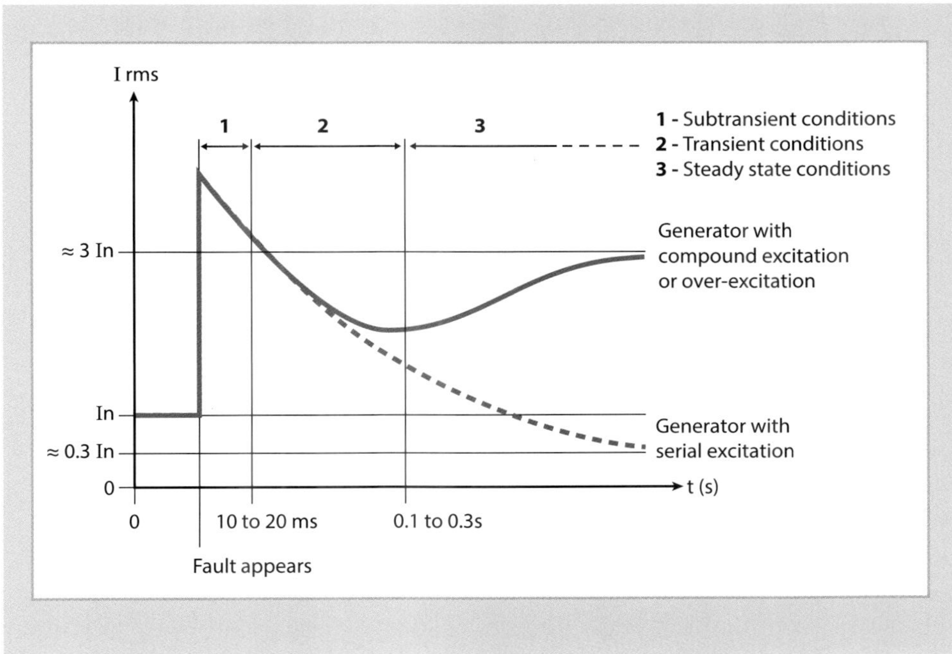

In reality, most sets are configured to combat this and the automatic voltage regulator affects the excitation, which brings the output of the generator up to approximately 3 times the output rating of the generator. Most healthcare generators recover to this level of output and can usually deliver this output from t=5 s to t=20 s before shutting down.

Appendix

Supplementary Information

4

A4.1 Extracts From Annex A of BS EN 60601-1:2006 + A1:2013

The extract below is supplied as supplementary information for the designer who wishes to push their design to explore the limits of the standards and not be restricted by the empirical solutions provided in most guidance.

A4.1.1 Touch current

The limits of 100 µA for normal conditions and 500 µA for single fault conditions are based on the following considerations.

The current density created at the heart by current entering the chest is 50 µA/mm² per ampere. The current density at the heart for 500 µA entering the chest is 0,025 µA/mm², which is well below the level of concern.

Touch current could conceivably reach an intra-cardiac site if careless procedures are used when handling intra-cardiac conductors or fluid filled catheters. Such devices should always be handled with great care and always with dry rubber gloves. The following risk analysis is based on pessimistic assumptions about the degree of care exercised.

The probability of a direct contact between an intra-cardiac device and an ME equipment enclosure is considered to be very low, perhaps 1 in 100 medical procedures. The probability of an indirect contact via the medical staff is considered to be somewhat higher, say 1 in 10 medical procedures. The maximum allowable leakage current in normal conditions is 100 µA, which itself has a probability of inducing ventricle fibrillation of 0.05. If the probability of indirect contact is 0.1, the overall probability is 0.005. Although this probability would appear undesirably high, it should be recalled that, with correct handling of the intra-cardiac device, this probability can be reduced to that for mechanical stimulation alone, which is 0.001.

The probability of the touch current rising to the maximum allowable level of 500 µA (single fault condition) is considered to be 0.1 in departments with poor maintenance (service) procedures. The probability of this current causing ventricular fibrillation is taken as 1. The probability of accidental contact directly with the enclosure is, as above, considered as 0.01 giving an overall probability of 0.001, equal to the probability of mechanical stimulation alone.

The probability of touch current at the maximum allowable level of 500 µA (single fault condition) being conducted to an intra-cardiac device by medical staff is 0.01 (0.1 for the single fault condition, 0.1 accidental contact). Since the probability of this current causing ventricular fibrillation is 1, the overall probability is also 0.01. Again, this probability is high, however, it can be brought down to the mechanical stimulation probability of 0.001 by adequate medical procedures.

A4.1.2 Patient leakage current – CF-type applied parts

The allowable value of patient leakage current for ME equipment with CF-type applied parts in normal conditions is 10 μA, which has a probability of 0.002 for causing ventricular fibrillation or pump failure when applied through small areas to an intra-cardiac site.

Even with zero current, it has been observed that mechanical irritation can produce ventricular fibrillation. A limit of 10 μA is readily achievable and does not significantly increase the risk of ventricular fibrillation during intra-cardiac procedures.

The 50 μA maximum allowed in single fault condition for ME equipment with CF-type applied parts is based on a value of current that has been found, under clinical conditions, to have a very low probability of causing ventricular fibrillation or interference with the pumping action of the heart.

For catheters with a diameter of 1.25 mm – 2 mm that is likely to contact the myocardium, the probability of 50 μA causing ventricular fibrillation is near 0.01. Small cross-sectional area (0.22 mm^2 and 0.93 mm^2) catheters used in angiography have higher probabilities of causing ventricular fibrillation or pump failure if placed directly on sensitive areas of the heart.

The overall probability of ventricular fibrillation being caused by patient leakage current in single fault conditions is 0.001 (0.1 for probability of single fault conditions, 0.01 probability of 50 μA causing ventricular fibrillation), equal to the probability for mechanical stimulation alone.

The 50 μA current allowed in single fault conditions is neither likely to result in a current density sufficient to stimulate neuromuscular tissues nor, if via direct current, cause necrosis.

A4.1.3 Patient leakage current – B- and BF-type applied parts

For ME equipment with B-type applied parts and BF-type applied parts, where the maximum allowable patient leakage current is 100 μA under normal conditions and 500 μA under single fault conditions, the same rationale applies as for touch current, since this current will not flow directly to the heart. (When applied parts of the same type are connected together higher limits are allowed of 500 μA in normal and 1000 μA in single fault conditions.) A limit of 5000 μA is allowed for BF applied parts when caused by an external voltage appearing on the connection.

The leakage current from applied parts on the surface of the body flows in a distributed manner through the body.

In the worst case situation, 5000 μA entering the chest would produce a current density at the heart of 0.025 μA/mm^2, well below the level for concern. Although this current would be perceivable by the patient the probability of occurrence is very small.

Appendix 5
Example risk assessment

▼ **Figure A5.1** Example risk assessment format

MEDICAL LOCATION ASSESSMENT/DESIGN STATEMENT

Client Name			Project Name / Address		Measures Agreed Y/N	Design Initials	Clinical Initials	Director Initials
A710 Rating	**Room description:** Detailed description of room use	Compliant	**Comments**		**Agreed Rating**			
Reg No/ Clause No	**Description of regulation**	Y/N	**Comments including clinical reasons**		Measures Agreed Y/N	Designer Signature/Initials	Clinicians Signature/Initials	Director Signature/Initials
	Detail of departure or requirement		Mitigation details					

POST CONSTRUCTION ASSESSMENT

Reg No/ Clause No	Description of regulation	Y/N	Comments including clinical reasons			
	Detail of departure or requirement		Mitigation details/implemented			
Review Date:		Review observations/actions Any significant changes since design agreed?				

Appendix
Typical medical IT system loads

6

A6.1 Typical medical IT system loadings

Cardiac theatre	7 kVA/Theatre
Thoracic theatre	5 kVA/Theatre
General theatre	2.5 kVA/Theatre
Cardiac intensive care	3 kVA/Bed
General recovery	2.5 kVA/Bed
Neonatal unit	3 kVA/Bed
ENT theatres	5 kVA/Theatre
Paediatric theatres	5 kVA/Theatre
Paediatric ICU	3 kVA/Bed

The above list is a guide for a designer to review and make their own decision about the load to be placed and the level of diversity to be applied when selecting a medical IT system.

Although these figures are quoted for loading purposes, it is vitally important that the designer takes into account the type of equipment used, how it is used and what other equipment is used in conjunction with it.

This will involve an assessment of a number of parameters which will include enclosure temperature, cable loading, conductor operating temperature and equipment characteristics such as starting current, in-rush current and harmonics. All of these factors will affect the selection of the protective device and the cable size.

A Guide to Electrical Installations in Medical Locations

Appendix

Thermal effects on circuit-breakers

7

Designers and installers should be aware of the effects of temperature on MCBs.

Table A7.1 contains the temperature correction values for circuit-breakers to BS EN 60898, indicating the reduction in rating against the temperature experienced in the enclosure.

▼ **Table A7.1** BS EN 60898 circuit breaker temperature correction values (courtesy of Hager)

Miniature circuit breaker
Standard EN 60898
Curve B, C and D

I_n (A)	-25 °C	-20 °C	-15°C	-10°C	-5 °C	0 °C	5 °C	10°C	15°C	20°C	25°C	30°C	35°C	40°C	45°C	50°C	55°C	60°C
6	8.64	8.4	8.16	7.92	7.68	7.44	7.2	6.96	6.72	6.48	6.24	6	5.76	5.52	5.28	5.04	4.8	4.56
10	14.4	14	13.6	13.2	12.8	12.4	12	11.6	11.2	10.8	10.4	10	9.6	9.2	8.8	8.4	8	7.6
13	18.7	18.2	17.7	17.2	16.6	16.1	15.6	15.1	14.6	14.0	13.5	13	12.5	12.0	11.4	10.9	10.4	9.9
15	21.6	21	20.4	19.8	19.2	18.6	18	17.4	16.8	16.2	15.6	15	14.4	13.8	13.2	12.6	12	11.4
16	23.0	22.4	21.8	22.1	20.5	19.8	19.2	18.6	17.9	17.3	16.6	16	15.4	14.7	14.1	13.4	12.8	12.2
20	28.8	28	27.2	26.4	25.6	24.8	24	23.2	22.4	21.6	20.8	20	19.2	18.4	17.6	16.8	16	15.2
25	36	35	34	33	32	31	30	29	28	27	26	25	24	23	22	21	20	19
32	46.1	44.8	43.5	42.2	41.0	39.7	38.4	37.1	35.8	34.6	33.3	32	30.7	29.4	28.2	26.9	25.6	24.3
40	57.6	56	54.4	52.8	51.2	49.6	48	46.4	44.8	43.2	41.6	40	38.4	36.8	35.2	33.6	32	30.4
50	-	-	-	-	-	62	60	58	56	54	52	50	48	46	44	42	40	38
63	-	-	-	-	-	-	-	-	-	-	-	63	60.5	58.0	55.4	52.9	50.4	47.9

In addition to the above enclosure, ambient temperature is should also be considered when groups of protective devices are loaded. Table A7.2 indicates the effect of groups of devices being loaded.

▼ **Table A7.2** Circuit-breaker grouping factors (courtesy of Hager)

Rated current reduced by factor K

Consideration should also be given to the proximity heating effect of the breakers themselves when fully loaded and mounted together in groups. There is a certain amount of watts loss from each breaker depending on the trip rating which may well elevate the ambient air temperature of the breaker above the ambient air temperature of the enclosure.

No. of units n	K (grouping factor)
$n = 1$	1
$2 \leq n < 4$	0.95
$4 \leq n < 6$	0.9
$6 \leq n$	0.85

Note: If the design current of a circuit (I_b) is less than 0.85 times the nominal setting of the circuit breaker (I_n) grouping can be ignored.

A group of 6 20 A MCBs in a cabinet where I_b is 17.5 A with an ambient temperature of 45 °C can be rated as follows:

I_n (Resultant) $= I_n$ (enclosure temp) × Factor K

Using the table values above:

I_n (enclosed temperature) $= 17.6$ A

As I_b of 17.5 A is more than 85 % of the I_n setting the factor K of 0.85 applies.

This gives a resultant I_n (resultant) of 17.6 A × 0.85 $= 14.96$ A

This is a significant reduction in I_n value and in this instance will be the difference between the protective device operating and staying operational. As can be seen if the design current is less than 85 % of the circuit breaker setting (I_n) then that group rating can be ignored.

A group of 6 20 A MCBs in a cabinet where all circuits are loaded in excess of 85 % but on the selected circuit I_b is 15.75 A with an ambient temperature of 45 °C can be rated as follows:

Using the table values above:

I_n (enclosed temperature) $= 17.6$ A

As the design current I_b of 17.75 A is less than 85 % of the I_n setting the factor K of 0.9 applies.

This gives a resultant I_n (resultant) of 17.6 A x 0.9 $= 15.84$ A

Therefore, in this instance this value is acceptable but the impact of grouping and ambient temperature have significantly affected the resultant value of I_n of the device.

Appendix 8

Effects of inrush current

An important factor when designing any circuit, but particularly final socket-outlet circuits, for theatre is to ensure that the effects of inrush are considered.

This phenomenon needs to be considered as the amount of medical equipment used in theatres is connected via an isolation transformer.

Traditionally, 20 A Type B MCBs have been used extensively. However, it has emerged that a number of events involving operation of the over-current protective device has occurred in theatre. Current assessments indicate that these trips are related to inrush current operating the circuit-breaker with the Type B time current curves.

In order to minimize these instances, designers of installations should ensure that the protective devices are selected to take into account the effects of a non-fault condition that would include the inrush from medical equipment transformers etc.

▼ **Figure A8.1** Transformer inrush effect (courtesy of Hager)

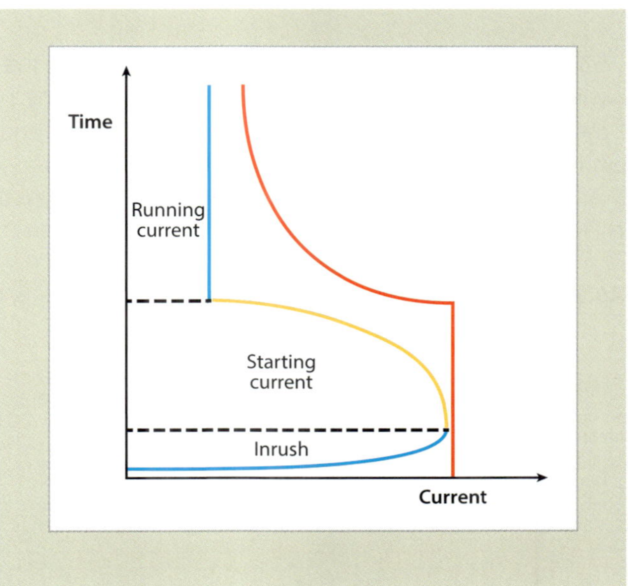

Figure A8.1 portrays the typical time current curves, demonstrating that inrush current is high for only a fraction of a second, for example, in the order of 0.2 s then falling significantly back to the steady state current value.

▼ **Table A8.1**   Transformer primary protective device ratings (courtesy of Hager)

Single Phase 230 V		Recommended MCB		
Transformer Rating (VA)	Primary Current	NBN	NCN	NDN
50	0.22	-	1	6
100	0.43	-	2	6
200	0.87	-	3	6
250	1.09	6	4	6
300	1.30	10	4	6
400	1.74	10	6	6
500	2.17	16	10	6
750	3.26	16	10	6
1000	4.35	25	16	10
2500	10.87	63	40	20
5000	21.74	-	63	32
7500	32.60	-	-	50
10000	43.48	-	-	63

Table A8.1 indicates the BEMA-recommended protective devices for the primary circuit of the transformer.

Regulation 533.2.1 requires designers to take account of the load under cyclic conditions which would include allowance for inrush from any piece of equipment. This would mean that the maximum inrush current from the equipment is less than the minimum instantaneous tripping current of the circuit-breaker serving the particular final circuit. An example of the effects of different values is sketched for illustration purposes in Figure A8.2.

▼ **Figure A8.2** Indicative inrush currents with respect to 20 A type, B, C and D curves

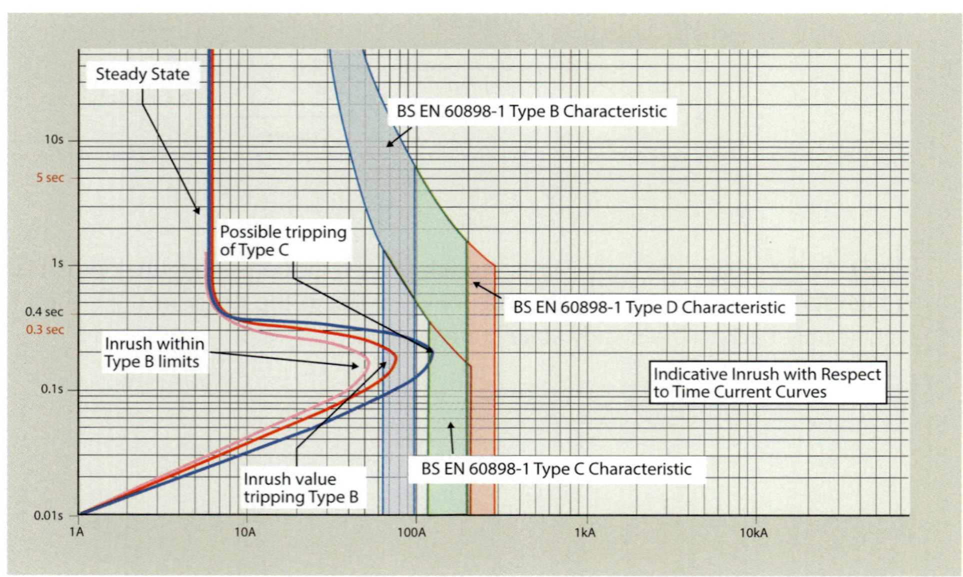

The following checklist is a suggested document for client organisations or those handing over Group 2 locations to use and develop for their own purposes:

BS 7671 Checklist – Group 2 Location

Hospital Name: _______________________________

Project Manager: _______________________________

Department/Room: _______________________________

Client Contact: _______________________________

General			
Cross out lines of items that are not applicable.		Date checklist conducted:	

Checklist			
	Yes	No	Comments
Confirmed with relevant staff the appropriate group rating for the location?	☐	☐	710.3
Identified any equipment requiring a TN (or TT) supply?	☐	☐	710.411.4. e.g. X-ray, cleaners and high power equipment etc.
Isolator & contactor control as required?	☐	☐	537. Also refer to equipment manufacturers installation instructions. Where frequent operation of high current (>50 A) isolators is required, contactor control should be used.
Automatic changeover of mains supply?	☐	☐	710.313.1 and 560.5
Sufficient RCD protected circuits are provided to prevent unwanted tripping due to normal leakage currents?	☐	☐	710.411.3.2.1 and 710.531.2.4. Fixed medical equipment may have 5 mA leakage per device so each supply may need individual protection.
RCD protection devices are only type A or type B and consideration has been given to the type fitted?	☐	☐	710.411.3.2.1. Refer to medical equipment manufacturer's installation instructions for guidance.

Checklist			
Wiring and protective devices meet disconnection times and simultaneously accessible voltage requirements?	☐	☐	710.411.3.2.5. This may require the resistance of protective conductors to be lower than the maximum values stated in 710.415.2.
Medical IT supply provided and meets requirements?	☐	☐	710.411.6. Also consider expected loading to ensure sufficient capacity for demand.
IT alarm system indicators easily visible and accessible from each protected location?	☐	☐	Staff using medical equipment needs to know if there is a fault in their location immediately.
Consideration given to installing a medical IT fault location system?	☐	☐	710.411.6.3.3. if No state reason:
Supplementary equipotential bonding provided, including sufficient connection points for medical equipment?	☐	☐	710.415.2.
EBB present and location appropriate ?	☐	☐	710.415.2.3.
Medical IT socket-outlets in patient environment un-switched, correctly marked and sufficient circuits?	☐	☐	710.553.1 If a light is fitted to indicate mains supply it should be green or a colour meeting BS EN 60601-1.
ELV supply for any fixed theatre lamp with appropriate autonomy?	☐	☐	710.560.6.1.1 A lamp used only for examination (as opposed to use in an operation) does not need to meet these requirements.
No mains or other cables in same containment as for medical system?	☐	☐	710.52 (710.444)
Medical equipment located in adjacent (control room) areas (Group 1) but connected to equipment in Group 2 has either IT or RCD supply?	☐	☐	710.1 Note 4 See medical equipment manufacturer's instructions.
Any illuminated room warning signs (X-rays on, laser on etc.) correctly installed and if not supplied by medical equipment have RCD protection?	☐	☐	710.444 Also consider EMI and in-rush currents as this may impact on the medical equipment.
Consideration given to EMI and EMC?	☐	☐	710.444. For example, medical equipment may be affected by static (e.g. disturbed ECG trace) so anti-static flooring may be required.

Testing			
	Pass	**Fail**	**Comments**
Electrical installation certified to BS 7671?	☐	☐	Check documents provided by electrical contractor.
Additional protection: Supplementary equipotential bonding installed correctly?	☐	☐	710.415.2 - Recorded as per 710.61 and 710.514.9
Supply impedance, phase & voltage correct for equipment to be installed?	☐	☐	Lower line impedance may be required than that required for automatic disconnection!
Medical IT system tests.	☐	☐	710.61 and Chapter 61
Contactor control, if fitted, works correctly?	☐	☐	Correct interlocking of start-stop buttons. Automatic re-start after supply loss (if fitted & providing no stop button pressed etc.).

Notes:

BS EN 60601 is the standard for any medical equipment used in the patient environment so covers items such as theatre lamps, ECG, ultrasound and X-ray equipment amongst other things. Testing of these devices should be with reference to BS EN 62353.

General Observations:

Actions:

ID	Action Item	Assigned To	Due By

Comments:

Checklist completed by:

Name: ____

Signature: _________________________________   **Date:** __/__/__

Tests conducted by:

Name: ____

Signature: _________________________________   **Date:** __/__/__

A Guide to Electrical Installations in Medical Locations

MEDICAL LOCATION TEST SHEET

Group No:

Project:		Job No:	
Address:		Date:	
Client:		Engine	

Room Name:		Test Instrument:	
Room No:		Serial Number:	
Room Loc:		Cal.Cert.No:	
Requested by:		Inspection Report No:	

Principal Tests	YES	NO	COMMENT
Is EBB located, terminated and Labelled as per BS 7671			
Are all mains power circuits ideally on the same phase and protected by a type A or B RCD.			
Has a minimum of 2 Medical IT Circuits been installed			
Are sockets/switches at least 200mm from medical gas outlets?			

	Circuit Details	AC TEST CURRENT					DC TEST CURRENT				
		$0.5x\ I_{\Delta n}$	$I_{\Delta n}$ (+ve)	$I_{\Delta n}$ (-ve)	$5x\ I_{\Delta n}$ (+ve)	$5x\ I_{\Delta n}$ (-ve)	$0.5x\ I_{\Delta n}$	$I_{\Delta n}$ (+ve)	$I_{\Delta n}$ (-ve)	$5x\ I_{\Delta n}$ (+ve)	$5x\ I_{\Delta n}$ (-ve)
Cct A											
Cct B											
GP Cct											
IT cct1											
IT cct2											

Item	Test item recorded clockwise from door	Max Z design	Z point to	Z point to EBB	IT alarm function	IT alarm leakage	PASS	FAIL
1	Cleaners socket							
2	General TN socket							
3	Light switches							
PENDANT 1								
4	Pendant body							
5	Structural steel							
IPS CCT 1/1								
6	SKT 1							
7	SKT 2							
8	SKT 3							
9	SKT 4							
10	SKT 5							
11	Oxygen							
12	Medical air							
IPS CCT 2/1								
13	SKT 1							
14	SKT 2							
15	SKT 3							
16	SKT 4							
17	SKT 5							
18	Vacuum							
19	Supplementary bonding points (LHS)							
20	Supplementary bonding points (RHS)							
21	Sink taps							
22	X-ray socket							
23	Drugs cupboard							
24	Radiator							
25	End of list							

Periodic Inspection and Testing- Annual measurements should be carried out to verify the resistance of the supplementary equipotential bonding is within the limits as required by the original design and BS 7671
This sheet should be appended to the relevant model form to provide supplementary information required by Section 710

The frequency of periodic inspection is addressed in BS 7671:2008+A3:2015 by two separate regulations, 622.1 and 622.2.

A11.1 Regulation 622.1: frequency of periodic inspections

Regulation 622.1 states:

"The frequency of periodic inspection and testing of an installation shall be determined having regard to the type of installation and equipment, its use and operation, the frequency and quality of maintenance and the external influences to which it is subjected. The results and recommendations of the previous report, if any, shall be taken into account."

A11.2 Regulation 622.2: alternative approach to periodic inspection

BS 7671:2008+A3:2015 allows an alternative approach to periodic inspection. Regulation 622.2 states:

"In the case of an installation under an effective management system for preventive maintenance in normal use, periodic inspection and testing may be replaced by an adequate regime of continuous monitoring and maintenance of the installation and all its constituent equipment by skilled persons, competent in such work. Appropriate records shall be kept."

Even though a hospital will normally be under the strict control of the maintenance provider, this approach is not ideal for the whole hospital installation as the 'effective management system' may be too difficult to achieve.

> **Note:** This does not preclude the use of new innovative processes under test at the time of publication.

Consequently, in order to determine a practical and workable approach to periodic inspection, wider considerations should be made.

Regulation 710.62 of BS 7671:2008+A3:2015 does not provide normative requirements as it consists only of notes. Note 1 to that Regulation sets out additional information particular to certain medical locations. Consequently, as there are some tasks that appertain to different types of medical locations, it would be more appropriate to separate out the installation types as detailed below. The maximum period between inspections should relate to the general fixed wiring with the additional requirement relevant to the location indicated in the notes.

As hospitals and healthcare premises are under strict maintenance regimes, the period between fixed wiring inspections could be extended if the specific requirements for the location are addressed in line with the frequencies recommended in Regulation 710.62. Table A11.1 below gives suggested frequencies.

▼ **Table A11.1** Recommended frequencies of inspection — medical locations

Type of installation	Routine check	Maximum period between inspections and testing	Note
Hospitals and medical clinics			
Hospitals and medical clinics: Group 0	1 year	5 years	-
Hospitals and medical clinics: Group 1	6 months	5 years	b
Hospitals and medical clinics: Group 2	6 months	5 years	a, b, c

Notes:

(a) Annually — complete functional tests of the insulation monitoring devices (IMDs)associated with the medical IT system including insulation failure, transformer high temperature, overload, discontinuity and the audible/visual alarms linked to them.

(b) Annually — measurements to verify that the resistance of the supplementary equipotential bonding is within the limits stipulated by Regulation 710.415.2.2.

(c) Every 3 years — measurements of leakage current of the output circuit and of the enclosure of the medical IT transformers in no-load condition, as specified by Regulation 710.512.1.1(i).

Index

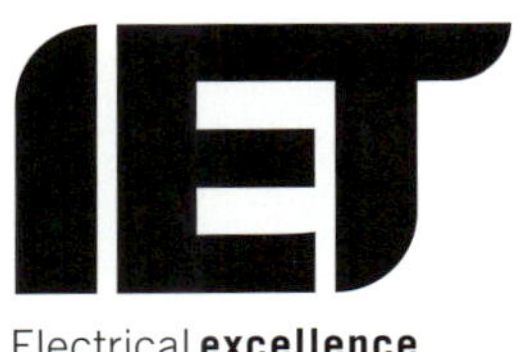

Expert publications

The IET is co-publisher of BS 7671 (IET Wiring Regulations), the national standard to which all electrical installations should conform. The IET also publishes a range of expert guidance supporting the Wiring Regulations.

You can view our entire range of titles including...

- BS 7671
- Guides
- Guidance Notes series
- Inspection, Testing and Maintenance titles
- City & Guilds textbooks and exam guides

...and more at:

www.theiet.org/electrical

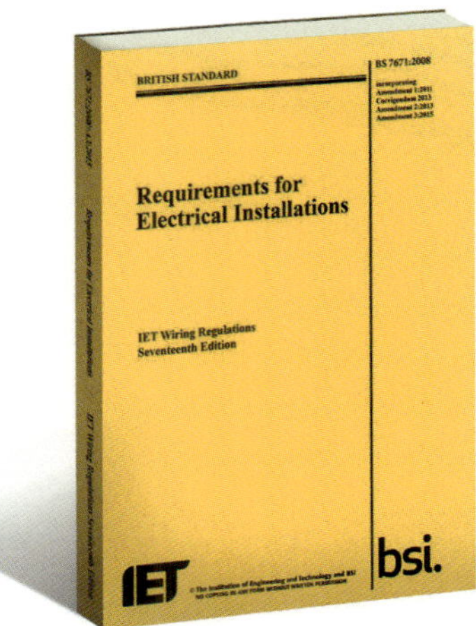

ELECTRICAL STANDARDS 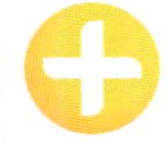

Constantly up-to-date digital subscriptions

Our expert content is also available through a digital subscription to the IET's Electrical Standards Plus platform. A subscription always provides the newest content, giving peace of mind that you are always working to the latest guidance.

It also lets you spread the cost of updating all your books once new versions are released.

Going digital gives you greater flexibility when working with the Wiring Regulations, Guidance Notes and the IET's expert Codes of Practice available for electrical engineers. The intuitive search function instantly serves results from across all books in your package. You can also access the content on your desktop, laptop or tablet, making it easy to take the content out on site or read on the move.

Find out more about our subscription packages and choose one to suit you at:

www.theiet.org/esplus